Love Your Sober Year

Kate Baily &
Mandy Manners

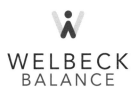

WELBECK
BALANCE

Published in 2022 by Welbeck Balance
An imprint of Welbeck Trigger Ltd
Part of Welbeck Publishing Group
Based in London and Sydney
www.welbeckpublishing.com

Design and layout © Welbeck Trigger Ltd 2022
Text © Kate Baily and Mandy Manners 2022
Illustrations © Amy Brazier 2022

A CIP catalogue record for this book is available from the British Library.

ISBN
Trade Paperback – 978-1-80129-071-5

Design by Alexandra Allden
Printed and bound in Dubai

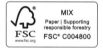

For the women of the Love Sober
Community and for you, reading this
book and making the brave and
brilliant choice to question
your relationship with alcohol.

CONTENTS

ABOUT THE AUTHORS

Kate Baily and Mandy Manners are sobriety and wellbeing coaches and habit change specialists who enable women to feel empowered by their choice to stop drinking alcohol. They use practical techniques and a holistic approach to growth, mindset and wellbeing to help women create successful sustainable sober living and to thrive in all areas of their lives.

In 2019 they co-founded Love Sober to provide coaching, online courses and a community for sober curious women. Their first book, *Love Yourself Sober: A Self Care Guide to Alcohol-Free Living for Busy Mothers*, was published in 2020. They also train coaches in Addictive Behaviours for The Coaching Academy.

Kate is an ICF accredited Life and Personal Performance Coach, and holds certificates in counselling, positive psychology and The Science of Happiness. A lifelong advocate of wellness and positive psychology she formalized her decades of self-study, moving from journalism into coaching in 2019. Kate lives in West Sussex with her husband, two children, dog, guinea pigs and chickens.

Mandy is a Certified Professional Recovery and Life Coach, member of the International Association of Professional Recovery Coaches and Trauma Informed Recovery Coach. She is a Mental Health First Aider and is studying for a Diploma in Fusion Therapeutic Coaching. Mandy lives in France with her husband, two children, cat and dog.

Lovesober.com
@lovesober.cic
@lovesoberpod
lovesoberpodcast

INTRODUCTION

For many of us, the journey to freedom from a toxic relationship with booze has been anything but straightforward. We have been back and forth, trapped in a negative cycle of drinking, feeling ashamed and vowing to never drink again – and then doing it again. Repeat ad infinitum. When we weren't drinking, we entered an upward spiral, when everything would slot into place. We would feel better, have more energy and better sleep. But then, life would throw a curveball our way, or we would forget the misery of hangovers and hit the F*** It button, and the negative drink cycle would start all over again.

We became fascinated with cycles, negative and positive. We searched for tools to empower us and keep us on the upward spiral. We asked ourselves how we could use the natural ebb and flow of our daily lives, our monthly cycles and our seasonal patterns, and work with our needs instead of overriding them. We searched for ways to flip from having negative self-talk, self-neglect, burnout and habitual drinking running the show to having self-care, self-love and balance at the heart of our lives. We asked ourselves: How can we create a framework to build a life we love sober? This book is how.

We fell in love with the seasons and natural rhythms we saw in the world around us. We noticed daily cycles, as day flows into night and night flows into day, touched by the transition spaces of dawn and dusk. We saw monthly cycles and seasons, as summer ebbed to winter and winter flowed to summer through autumn and spring. We witnessed the way we experience our life cycles from puberty to motherhood to menopause.

We found our process of breaking free from the clutches of alcohol also followed a cyclical pattern and were fascinated to find that this was echoed by models in psychology, which we will be looking at in each season in the book.

We also focus on the upward spiral of change that comes from the decision to be alcohol-free and, using the ideas in these models, we have developed a cyclical methodology for sustainable sobriety to support this – our R4 Balance Method works with the delicate balance needed between action and reflection, innovation and rest to honour the cycles of growth and wellbeing that ensure successful and satisfying sober living. Relating to the seasons, this method gives each part of the year a focus, as follows:

Restore – Spring: growth and preparation, restoring the foundations of our sobriety and wellbeing. Setting our intentions for future action.

Reignite – Summer: conservation and action, reigniting the passion and purpose in our sober journey while protecting our needs and respecting our boundaries.

Rewrite – Autumn: release and maintenance, rewriting the story of our habits and behaviour and developing sustainable tools for living well, free from alcohol.

Rest – Winter: reorganization and contemplation, resting in order to integrate wisdom learnt from the previous cycles to nurture ourselves and our sober-selves and allow for future growth.

This has been designed with reference to two theoretical models that marry the wisdom of seasonal living with the cycles of the sober journey. The first model, the Panarchic theory[1], is based on universal patterns we see in the seasons that underpin evolution and resilience. It follows the familiar journey of the year: growth in spring, conservation in summer evolving to release in autumn before completing the cycle with winter's role of integration and reorganization . . . Then the wheel turns again.

---

1 Gunderson, L & Holling, CS (2018). *Panarchy Theory*. Available at: www.resalliance.org

The second model, *The Stages of Change* by Prochaska and DiClemente[2], is a fundamental model for understanding behaviour and addiction. Sober-curiosity begins in the cold fallows of our sober 'winter', as we reflect on our relationship with alcohol and come to the realization that change is necessary. We call this period of time 'contemplation'.

We then enter the preparation stage in our first sober 'spring', getting onboard what we need to make change happen. Next comes the cycle of action where we cultivate the energy of our 'summer' to make changes. After this we enter the maintenance stage in 'autumn' to contemplate our further growth in the rest period of winter. These are our sober seasons, if you like.

By tuning in to nature and to our solar seasons and cycles we can rebalance wellbeing in a long-term and sustainable way and stave off the Wine Witch (the Addictive Voice) – that nagging inner critic telling us one glass won't hurt – in line with these universal principles.

In this book you will find weekly tools and strategies to underpin your wellbeing, help you manage stress and booze triggers, harness your creativity and find the kind of sober self-care menu that makes you feel like you have come home. By building your sober toolkit, you will have the skills and practices to pace yourself, manage your expectations and challenge limiting beliefs. We have also included other cyclical models, in the third week of each season, such as the habit loop and the change cycle. Trust us, once you start seeing cycles, you will find them everywhere!

When we decide to stop drinking it can feel like a cold hard stop, an empty space that feels both uncomfortable and intolerable – a bit like winter. We are not unlike new farmers with empty fields and no idea what to sow in them, no clue what size they are nor what they are capable of growing. Once we have cleared this space, however, we can attend to the quiet growth of our sober journey, looking after ourselves day in and day out. We have planted the seed and as these patterns become new habits, signs of life appear. We see shoots of possibility as we enter our RESTORE season of growth. Our sober spring has arrived. Like crops thriving with water and nutrients, we can feel a surge of energy and a sense of what may just be possible.

As we head into our sober summer, the REIGNITE part of our cycle, our sobriety matures slightly. We enter the static haze of summer, which can be a beautiful mellowing

2   Prochaska, J & DiClemente, C (1994). *The Transtheoretical Approach: Crossing Traditional Boundaries of Therapy*. Krieger Publishing Company.

time as we let the warmth fortify us for deeper work and the inevitable storm clouds ahead. We learn that we need to pace ourselves and adjust to the bigger cycles at work. There could be feelings of flatness, and therefore doubt, creeping in every three months in a cyclical way. We must conserve the sober momentum.

The summer can also coincide with busy times and holidays, and we can run ourselves ragged, forget the early lessons and find ourselves triggered to drink again, tempted by hedonistic impulses and quick fixes rather than stopping to connect with our overarching wellness and long-term goals.

As the sun passes its zenith and the days grow shorter, we are really reaping some benefits from sowing our sober intentions and seeds. We enjoy better sleep, our moods have levelled, and we are feeling more confident and established in our sobriety. We have hit milestones and really started to change old patterns and rewire neural pathways. The grasshopper has sung all summer and now we are turning inward to autumn. We are into the REWRITE phase of our R4 Balance cycle.

We need the darkening days after the light days of summer. This REWRITE part of the cycle affords us time to reflect and reminds us – with the falling leaves – of what we can let go, what no longer serves us. Once released, these feelings can mulch down and be repurposed to feed new growth and new ideas. Autumn is a great time for getting our nurturing shoes on and kicking through the leaves. We have another equinox to remind us of the balance of light and dark, that it's OK to feel sad and to be with our feelings, and honour our darkness and loss as well as celebrate the good times.

Lastly, we head into winter, our season of REST. In this time of our sobriety, it's a time to reflect, to take stock of how far we have come. We reintegrate and reorganize at this time of year. We may have big festivals or holidays and once again, overwhelm can rear its head. As a static season, like summer, we are encouraged by the wisdom of nature to take a more passive role, to rest as much as we can. This is the field lying fallow to allow for restoration in spring, this is the night to our day and the rest to our activity. It is the perfect season to reflect on what we have done well, what we have accomplished, and feel proud of ourselves before we rush into making new wishes and new resolutions.

When we stop drinking, in whichever season in whichever year we do this, we need new resources – tools to help us cope with the stressors of our lives. It's strange to think of alcohol as a resource, but it's helpful in this context to look at it as a negative resource but a resource, nonetheless. We want to encourage you to cultivate and discover new positive resources internally (such as self-compassion, boundaries, resilience) and externally (such as routines, timetables, supportive rituals, sober treats). We can use these as a scaffold while our bodies and minds heal and the internal resources are built and strengthened. Time and repetition are the key, which is why using a timetable of the natural year can be so helpful. It's there for us and has worked for humans for millennia. Instead of drinking to calm down at the end of the day, to get us through the time of the month or to override our flagging energy levels, we can use these new resources to live better, feel better and stay better.

HOW TO USE THIS BOOK

This book is designed for you to use however you wish. You might want to start at the beginning and work through the seasons from your own sober starting point, beginning with the spring section, whatever the time of year. Or you could journey alongside the actual seasons, so your outside environment mirrors the season and chimes with the work you are doing in the book – it is a cyclical process, after all, so you will reach all seasons eventually. Finally, you might choose to dip into any one of the seasons at any time, should you ever feel you need its tone, tools and essence.

Each time we head into a different season we are influenced by the elements, cultural influences and family legacies associated with that season. All of these can be potential triggers, but also potential areas of growth and reclamation. In each season, we provide a planner template to help you to put your best foot forward and avoid any potholes on your sober path.

Each week also contains journaling prompts to help you deepen your exploration of the topics and your journey through them. We recommend you choose a lovely journal for yourself and create a ritual for your journaling, such as a favourite time of the week. Work through the questions and note any further reflections as you wish, and decorate it as you would like. Make it your own and special to you. Use it as a little sacred space for you to work with your *Love Your Sober Year* book.

We hope you enjoy this journey through the seasons and exploration of how the awareness of cycles within your own life can support your wellbeing and nurture your choice to be alcohol-free.

Spring

'I dwell in possibility.'
EMILY DICKINSON

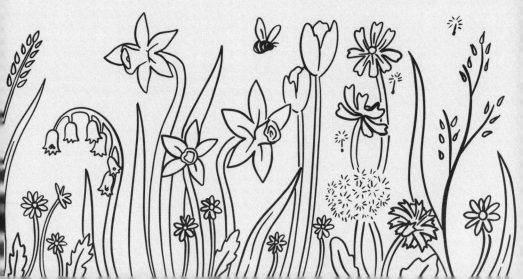

HARNESSING THE POWER OF THE GIFTS OF SPRING TO RESTORE

Spring is associated with new beginnings, new ideas, optimism and rebirth. We see the first bulbs appear, alongside baby animals, and sense the lengthening days more palpably. In sober circles, people often experience the beginning of their sober journey as a honeymoon period with its attendant feelings of invincibility and lust for life. Like boisterous toddlers finding our feet, we need support around us and an environment that helps us to learn this new way of living. We need to clear away obstacles and reduce risks, being mindful not to run before we can walk. In coaching, this is the start of a virtuous upward spiral where we set out our goals and intentions for the beginning of our journey.

Early sober spring is a delicate balance of both heady optimism and steady routine. We need a good deal of hope and optimism at this stage as we may toil without obvious fruition or reward, as much of the work we are doing is underground. Preparing the right conditions will bring dividends if we show up each day and make a pillow promise to hit the hay without having drunk alcohol.

As we grow into our sobriety, a bulb shoots and begins to grow. We need to nurture its roots to protect its growth, tending carefully to the basics of our routines and being patient with ourselves. Spring is about RESTORING our health, reconnecting with things we loved before alcohol got in the way and preparing the ground for sober growth. In late spring, the shoots begin to appear and we pick up some momentum. Day in and day out, we build habits, seeing shoots of possibility, and the upward spiral starts to have a life of its own. We find sober friends, and the time we have regained from drinking – and recovering from drinking – is filled with hobbies, learning, resting, and our healing journey begins to flower.

Spring is a special time, vulnerable yet steely in determination. We know we can't control everything but by setting the intention to change our relationship with alcohol we know what we are planting and what we want to grow and manifest in our lives. Now we just need to practice daily self-care to cultivate favourable conditions for our sobriety to blossom.

The key themes we are going to explore in spring are:

- Setting intentions, growth, new ideas, optimism, inspiration, changing habits, managing stress triggers, overcoming people-pleasing, and nurturing self-care

Return to spring any time you feel the need to reset intentions or revisit the groundwork you have already laid.

REASONS TO BE CHEERFUL IN SPRING

Daffodils, bulbs, eggs, baby animals, new exercise, new journal, spring cleaning, Easter eggs, blossom, nature trails, hope, wishes, new plans, optimism.

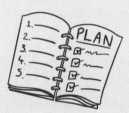 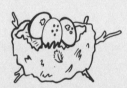 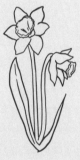

FOR YOUR JOURNAL

How do I want to feel this spring?

What matters to me the most this season?

What about this season makes me feel at my happiest/calmest /most joyful?

What would I like to create or nurture in my life this season?

What elements make spring special for me?

What fears would I like to release this spring?

Because I was sober, this week I . . .

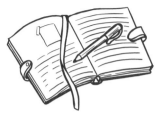

WEEK 1:
YOUR SEASONAL PLANNER

'Plan your work and work your plan.'
UNKNOWN

Before we dive in, let's have a look at the overview of your spring. Like seasonal cartographers, we design our life map according to the natural features and lay of the land and plan our route to better prepare for our journey. What celebrations do you have coming up? What challenges might they bring? Is it a heavy work season? How can you take things off the list? What fun things have you got to look forward to? None? Right. Let's fix that!

We always say that sober tools are life tools, in that they help us manage stress, find comfort, and identify what we authentically need to be well. Some of these are practices such as self-compassion or movement and some are practical tools to manage our time.

Here we have provided a simple planner to note your intentions for specific dates and some questions for deeper reflection to help you prepare for your Sober Spring.

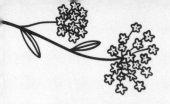

SPRING
Planner

Month 1

Month 2

Month 3

Hobbies to try ....
....
....

Key dates

Possible Triggers

Strategy..
Movement ....
Self-care ....

HOW TO USE YOUR PLANNER

Look through your diary and pick out the days that are family birthdays, major festivals or national bank holidays. Plan for when you will need to self-protect your sober choice the most.

Creating a life you love sober is about widening your choices and trying out new things. Your life may have revolved around alcohol for a long time – now it's time to flex your sober muscle and try new things. So, this season challenge yourself to:

- Choose a social activity that you want to try alcohol-free
- Try a new alcohol-free drink
- Have a go at a new hobby or activity that you have always wanted to try
- Say no to something you don't want to do
- Add in some movement (such as dancing or stretching)
- Practice self-care

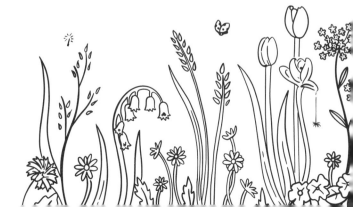

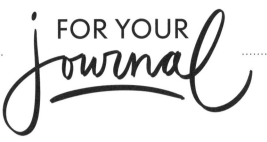

FOR YOUR Journal

What associations do I have with these major dates coming up?
How confident on a scale of 1-10 (1 being low confidence and
10 being watertight) do I feel about managing this period alcohol-free?
Which activities do I want to opt out of this year?

What key dates have I identified that are important to me?
How do they normally relate to drinking alcohol?
What new rituals can I introduce?
Are there certain dates I need to plan around because of alcohol?
What will I do?

What do I need to do to increase my confidence level by 1 point on these dates?
(Have a friend there, opt out, drive, journal more, get a coach?)
What might I do instead?
What might I drink instead?

What can I plan in instead?
Because I was sober, this week I . . .
What is your confidence level now out of 1–10? Hopefully it will have improved.
If not, go back and see if you can generate more options to encourage you.

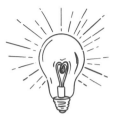

WEEK 2 :
SETTING YOUR INTENTION
Seed wishes

'Begin with the end in mind.'
JOHN WHITMORE

In coaching, rather than focusing on the problems right in front of us, we focus our attention by asking questions to get a clear picture of what we actually want, rather than what we simply don't want. If we can imagine a life free of hangovers, with boundless energy, better sleep and sparkling eyes, this is going to motivate us more in the long run than just thinking, 'I really don't want to drink'.

Although this coaching approach is a modern modality, it actually has its roots in ancient yogic traditions. At the beginning of new cycles, practitioners would use mantras called sankalpas or seed wishes – affirmations of positive intent – to help them align with what they wanted to bring to fruition.

The idea of the sankalpa is more than a resolution. Rather than something we are striving for, it is articulating a seed of possibility as if it is already true. ('I am happily sober', 'I am present', 'I have peace'.) The passing of time and the right conditions and care make the sankalpa grow and bear fruit. These wishes are set with self-compassion and acceptance. Although we want our plant to grow and bear fruit, it will take time, and there is nothing wrong with the seed if it has to be re-sown a few times to find the right growing conditions. New habits take time and practise and we are starting to embed our sober habit in this very first stage by naming our intention and making it explicit to ourselves. After we set our intention, we take small daily steps and trust the process. We have made a promise to ourselves and we can return to this seed wish and use it as an anchor to remember our intention.

When I decided to stop drinking the last time, I made a promise to myself that came out of a self-compassion practice which had a profound experience on me. I realized that when I drank alcohol, I disconnected from myself and I promised I would never abandon myself again. That morning, I wrote my sobriety mantra which is, 'Sobriety is my fundamental act of self-care, which informs all others.' Sankalpa actually means a "vow to your highest truth". Whatever the trigger or feeling that came my way over the next few weeks or months I went back to that mantra, which I couldn't argue with – it was just true. KATE

My sober seed wish was around mental health. I am doing the best I can to look after my brain. When I had the knowledge that alcohol made depression worse, I couldn't unknow that. I made a promise to do what I could to be well. I made the intention to live not taking my health for granted. I had brought children into the world and they deserved a better example, someone who modelled self-care, self-compassion and healed their own pain rather than hid from it. MANDY

WAYS TO WORK WITH SEED WISHES

Here are just a few ideas to get you started . . .

Create positive sober statements

Sit quietly and focus on your breath, then ask yourself, 'What is my deepest sober desire? What do I want sobriety to give me?' Then frame it as a positive statement. 'I am happily sober.' I am confident and content in alcohol-free living.'

Make some intention stones

Collect some smooth pebbles and write your seed wishes on them.

Plant some seeds

You can plant seeds at any time of the year and it can be very comforting and grounding. We can visualize the passing of time, and care for and nurture plants as a symbol of our sobriety.

Create intention art

Decorate your seed wish or create a collage around it. Engaging the creative side of your brain helps with habit change by making your new habit satisfying and visible.

Write a sobriety mantra

Again, this is your own personal mantra relating to your sober journey. Start with 'Sobriety is . . .' and add what it means to you. For example, 'Sobriety is . . . freedom, happiness, health, hearing myself, and self-care'. Write something that feels empowering, positive and personal to you. You can use this if you feel wobbly, or perhaps read it first thing every morning.

These are all ways we can work creatively to plant and nurture our sober intentions in satisfying and varied ways.

FOR YOUR *journal*

What do
I want?

What is the
promise I
am making
to myself?

How can I
nurture this first
step of sobriety?

What hopes and
wishes do I want
sobriety to give me?
Health?
Greater energy?

How will I
know when it
is working?

What will I gain
by getting sober
and creating a
life I can
love sober?

Because I was sober, this week I . . .

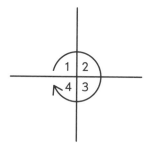

WEEK 3:
CYCLES AND SOBRIETY
The habit loop

'The first step to getting somewhere is to decide you are not going to stay where you are.'
ANON

Spring is a great time to adopt new habits. The symbology of the new year makes it popular for many of us to attempt habit change at this point as it feels like a great time to wipe the slate clean and start fresh after December 31st. But in keeping with the rhythms of the year, and spring being a time of new beginnings in nature, it makes sense for us to capitalize on this renewed energy and extra daylight to affect habit change. This comes a couple of months after New Year's Eve, for people in the Northern Hemisphere while, of course, spring starts around September if you are down under.

We are indeed creatures of habit and have survived successfully as a species partly because of habits. If you think about how many actions we take each day, if we had to consciously think about each one, we would never get anything done! We learn habits by forming a habit loop of memory - we perform Behaviour X, and this brings certain pleasurable results because dopamine is released in the brain. Because it feels nice, we repeat Behaviour X until it becomes habitual, unconscious or involuntary.

In his book, *Atomic Habits*, author James Clear breaks down the habit loop into four parts: cue, craving, response and reward. In the case of drinking alcohol, the loop might work as follows: cue = stress; craving = wanting a glass of wine; response = drinking the wine; reward = temporary numbness caused by alcohol. If we repeat this loop, we need to do it more and more over time and increase the quantity of the response as our brain adapts to anything we keep repeating, requiring more to reach the same result. Because alcohol unbalances our neurotransmitters, over time it ends up actually causing the stress, which only feeds and perpetuates the cycle.

The habit loop

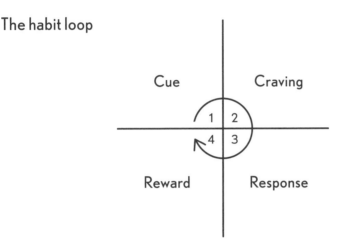

When alcohol consumption has crossed that line into habitual, problematic drinking, many people describe their relationship with it as being stuck in a hamster wheel. Albert Einstein reportedly said, 'Insanity is doing the same thing over and over again and expecting different results.' Is that how your drinking habit feels? It certainly did to us . . .

We now know from neuroscience and brain imaging that we can get addicted to anything, from online shopping to gambling to tattoos. The insidious thing about alcohol is it's the only addictive, mind-altering drug that is legal and positively encouraged. It is also one of the only drugs – along with opiates such as heroin – where withdrawal from it can cause death. We can't escape the ancient biology of our dopamine loopy brains but we can work with them to replace unhealthy habits with helpful and healthy ones, thereby unhooking ourselves from the bad ones, with repetition and a strategy.

I was literally so bored of having the same conversations with myself. I couldn't see a life without alcohol in it. My diaries are full of circular conversations and failed attempts at moderation. Every time I woke up feeling jaded and dehydrated after drinking, I would tell myself how much I hated it and decide to give up. Three days later, I felt better and would decide to have a glass of wine and the whole cycle would repeat again. Trying to control the amount, the type of alcohol, or make different rules around drinking was futile and kept me stuck, locked in this loop. The only way to stop the cycle was to remove alcohol. KATE

I had a very strong unconscious belief that I had to win at this battle with alcohol by 'managing' alcohol in my life. However, the more I let alcohol back in my life after quitting again, the less I liked myself and the less deserving I felt of positive change. In the end, I realized that turning towards, and not away from, being sober was the only choice I could make in my life. MANDY

Inspired by Clear's work, we suggest using these four steps to help break the negative habit of drinking alcohol:

1. Make it difficult – get rid of any booze from the house.
2. Make it invisible – come off social media except sober forums.
3. Make it unsatisfying – keep old diaries handy so it motivates you to not go back.
4. Make it unrewarding – be accountable by telling people on a sober forum that you want to stop drinking. They will offer support and encouragement, and being seen is super-helpful in keeping to your plan.

To build the new good habit of being sober, we then reverse the process by flipping the stages above into positive steps, like this:

1. Make it easy – buy some lovely AF (alcohol-free) drinks for your home.
2. Make it visible – perhaps create a vision board of sober celebs, and/or change the passwords on your computer to something like, 'I am a sober badass.'
3. Make it satisfying – read quit lit and inspiring sober posts
4. Make it rewarding – post day counts on sober forums and buy yourself some sober treats

Soon, your virtuous cycle will begin to turn and gather momentum – becoming, over time, your new unconscious habit. You will feel better and more sure-footed, able to cope to and build a variety of different responses to your stress cues – using your sober toolkit of exercise, treats, rewards, positive connections and rest.

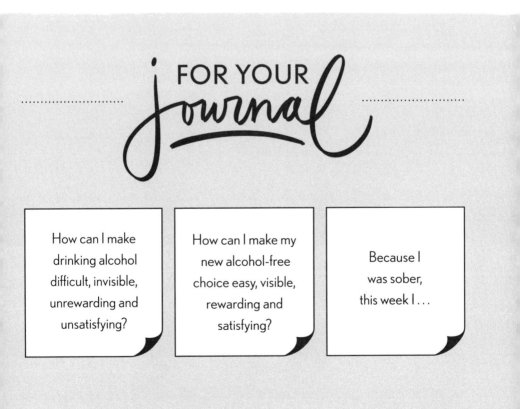

FOR YOUR Journal

| How can I make drinking alcohol difficult, invisible, unrewarding and unsatisfying? | How can I make my new alcohol-free choice easy, visible, rewarding and satisfying? | Because I was sober, this week I … |

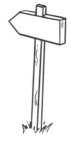

WEEK 4 :
CULTIVATING SOBER SPACE
Habit change

'Watch your thoughts, they become your words; watch your words, they become your actions; watch your actions, they become your habits; watch your habits, they become your character; watch your character, it becomes your destiny.'
LAO TZU

Many of us enter into sobriety with pretty strong motivation to change. We have had enough, it has become 'too much' or we have become so tired of letting ourselves down. However, after a while this resolve often fades and we fall back into old habits. We use willpower to not drink rather than creating a life we love sober. Think about how many times our new year's resolutions fall by the wayside after a couple of weeks. We cut out carbs or sugar, abstain from alcohol, usually focusing on the deprivation and gritting our teeth for long enough to feel a temporary improvement . . . and then back we go. Willpower alone does not work because, quite simply, it runs out.

It has been proven time and again that you cannot scare people into long-term habit change. We are educated with facts and statistics around smoking and cancer risks and yet, even knowing this, a lot of us smoked or still do. We did it because for us it represented something emotionally. If you grew up in the 80s and 90s, you only had to watch movies like *Grease* to develop an unconscious belief that to get the guy and be included, cool and sexy you had to ditch your twinset, get some leather – and smoke.

Putting it simply, we need the carrot and not just the stick. We need to create the right conditions, change our habits, our mindsets and our environments to generate sustainable habit change and over time, as we saw last week, the upward spiral and gather momentum.

There is a well-known analogy of the elephant, the rider and the path that is often used to explain habit change[3]. The rider is our left logical brain that makes decisions based on intellectual sense, logic and facts. The elephant is the emotional right side of our brain that makes decisions based on feelings and memory, and the path is our environment. When making a decision to change, there is no way the rider (logic) can force the elephant to change path (using willpower) because our emotions (the elephant) will always do what they want.

In order to change the mind of the elephant (our emotional connection to our behaviour), we have to clear the path (our environment) and make the new path feel good to the elephant. We have to have a really strong connection to the benefits we will get from our decision to change. We can use the rider to become informed – log on to a sober forum, generate actions and plans. We can engage the elephant by working with our values, reflections, future self and goals, and reward our progress with alcohol-free alternatives that feel good. We also need to work on the liminal thinking or unconscious messaging around alcohol (see page 78). Then we boss our environments by removing alcohol, getting support and, over time, our elephant will know the way to go.

Eventually, once we have repeated the action enough for it to become an automatic habit – we have engaged our elephant – we actually begin to 'feel' like a non-drinker, and then we start to think of ourselves as a sober person. We might be a Sober Dignified Woman, in the words of Tammi Salas, or a Sober Badass like Holly Whittaker, author of *Quit Like a Woman*, or a Sober Diva like RuPaul. The sober habit has become your action, your thought, your character and has changed your destiny.

---

3 Haidt, J (2007). *The Happiness Hypothesis*. Cornerstone

"We might be a Sober Dignified
Woman, in the words of Tammi Salas,
or a Sober Badass like Holly Whittaker,
author of *Quit Like a Woman*, or a
Sober Diva like RuPaul."

FOR YOUR
Journal

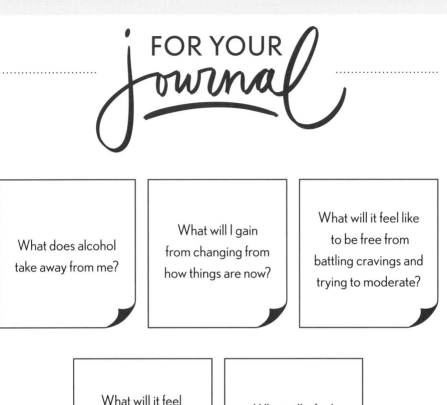

What does alcohol take away from me?

What will I gain from changing from how things are now?

What will it feel like to be free from battling cravings and trying to moderate?

What will it feel like to be free from shame around my drinking?

What will it feel like never to have a hangover again?

What does my 'free from alcohol' life look like?
What do I drink instead? What do I wear?
What hobbies do I have? How much money do I save?

Because I was sober, this week I . . .

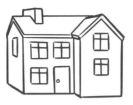

WEEK 5 :
BOSSING YOUR ENVIRONMENT
Stress triggers and sensory

*'The greatest gift of the garden is the
restoration of the five senses.'*
HANNA RION

We like to think of sobriety as a bit like having a sober garden makeover by Monty Don (UK garden expert, if you don't know him). Being sober takes work, like removing the bindweed that alcohol has wound around our lives, our occasions, associations and routines. It also takes maintenance and pruning and stopping to scratch our chins and to take a good look at what we want and need in our new lady garden (not THAT kind of lady garden).

We all have sensory needs and preferences. If we tune in to this part of our experience, it can provide brilliant information to enable us to soothe ourselves, leave triggering situations before it's too late and enable us to lower our stress response. Being skilled and intimate with our sensory needs is therefore a lethal weapon against the Wine Witch.

Do you feel stressed if things are too loud, or if three people are talking to you at once? (Hello, motherhood.) Perhaps you find it hard to relax if the room is too bright, or feel stressed in supermarket queues. Do scratchy labels drive you mad? Sensory needs are very real needs and certainly if you identify as being an HSP (Highly Sensitive

Person)[4] these can be significant reasons why you drank. We drank to make the room quieter, the world a little less busy and, essentially, to soothe a ragged nervous system when our senses were flooded. Once we stopped drinking, we were able to get in touch with our sensory needs and meet them authentically.

If we sprint and crash and ignore the sensory little red flags, the stress in our system builds throughout the day and, like a pressure cooker about to blow, we hit the F*** It button and reach for the wine. We used to ignore the feelings of tiredness building, of thirst or even of needing to go to the loo, then would crash and hit the wine at the end of the day.

The temporary numbness alcohol provides increases cortisol in the body and depletes neurotransmitters, which makes us less and less able to cope over time. So, we MUST slow down and replace that wine (or whatever your poison is) with HEALTHY resources. This way, we build the capacity of regulating our system gently and following our needs of thirst, hunger and tiredness or needing the loo, and this gentle awareness and the subsequent remedies or mini-actions act like oiling a bike chain to help it run smoothly through the gears.

You can balance sensory overwhelm by taking sensory breaks in order for you to calm your nervous system. Check out the table on the next page for some ideas of how to counterbalance overwhelm in your different senses. It's not just about dialing things down – it's about replacing stress triggers with alternatives you love and that soothe you. Respect the ebb to boss the flow.

Looking after my sensory needs is key to my sobriety. I realized, after I stopped drinking that I often drank to make things go quiet. I need lowlights and plenty of alone time. If I look after my sensory needs my mental health looks after itself, to be honest. KATE

Learning about my sensory needs has been a huge part of my sober toolkit: I am very triggered by noise, which is probably why I would head straight to the bar and down a drink to cope at a busy party. I am also sensitive to smell. I find it hard to settle if there are strong smells in my immediate environment. MANDY

---

4 Aron, E (2017). *Highly Sensitive Person*. Available at: hsperson.com

A sensory toolkit – things that help us to soothe ourselves

SENSE	TOOLS (These are some of our favourites, do add your own.)
Sight	Flames (fire/candles); a room with a view; flowers; trees; eye mask; sunglasses; sitting with your eyes closed in the sunshine; watching Netflix
Sound	Noise-cancelling headphones; binaural beats; birdsong
Smell	Essential oils (bergamot, bitter orange, lavender); cooking with spices; moisturizing lotion
Taste	Decaf Earl Grey; dark chocolate; spicy food; ginger
Touch	Blankets; stroking animals; cosy knits
Introception (internal organ sensations) This could be needing the toilet, being thirsty – any senses within the body we might ignore.	Early nights; remembering and answering to HALT triggers (Hungry, Angry, Lonely, Tired – see page 38)
Vestibular (balance/movement) This could be feeling dizzy or motion sick	Mini breaks throughout the day (even if it's just grabbing five minutes alone in the bathroom); sitting by the window at work; slowing down
Proprioceptive (sensations in our muscles and joints) This could be neck ache, back ache or clenched teeth, for example.	Massage; big scarves; hot-water bottle; heated blanket; weighted blanket; yoga

FOR YOUR journal

What are my sensory needs?

What are my sensory preferences?

Which ones have I been ignoring?

How can I slow down and authentically meet that need?

What resources have worked for me in the past?

How can I add them in to be helpful in my sober lifestyle?

How can I protect mini breaks throughout the day?

Because I was sober, this week I . . .

WEEK 6 :
RESEARCHING OUR RESOURCES
The magic of our nervous system

*'For me there is something primitively soothing about
this music, and it went straight to my nervous system,
making me feel ten feet tall.'*
ERIC CLAPTON

This week we add to the sensory toolkit of last week by looking carefully at our environments, our resources, the things that are available to us that give us comfort and safety and joy and excitement. Now we are starting to get really badass about working with our needs by exploring the science of our autonomic nervous system (ANS), which is the neurobiology of our fight/flight/freeze responses and how we can regulate and rest. This is an exercise to build awareness and use these gifts intentionally to change our emotional state. This may be new knowledge and, in the springtime we may be more open to trying new things and seeing things with fresh eyes – so be curious as you explore what makes *you* feel good.

The three states of the Autonomic Nervous System

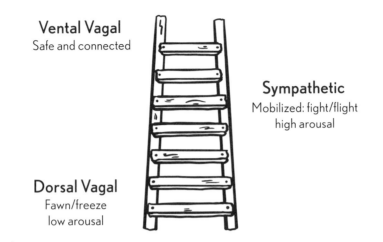

Vental Vagal
Safe and connected

Sympathetic
Mobilized: fight/flight
high arousal

Dorsal Vagal
Fawn/freeze
low arousal

The ideal states for us to live in for optimal health and wellbeing are a combination of the Ventral Vagal State (at the top of the ladder) where we feel safe and connected going about our daily business, and the Dorsal Vagal State (at the bottom of the ladder) where we rest and digest, in a state of low arousal, downing tools and stopping activity. If we face any kind of stressor or danger, we enter the Sympathetic State where we need to activate a survival response – such as fight, flight or freeze – for a short amount of time before returning to the Ventral Vagal State once the threat has passed and we have released the stress. (For more on the stress cycle see Week 9 in each season.)

If you are stressed and in fight, flight or freeze mode (anxious, sweaty palms, elevated heartbeat, on edge, angry, etc.) you are in the high arousal, Sympathetic State and need to calm down and/or release stress. If you are feeling blocked, stuck, bored or have low energy you may be in in low arousal Dorsal Vagal State, and you could benefit from something to pick you up or energize you. The ability to recognize, tap in to and control these responses is a super power, and helps us to get us out of the craving brain state and maintain our sobriety.

Firstly, we identify where we are on the ANS Ladder (see illustration). Then we can create a toolkit of resources – as polyvagal and trauma expert Deb Dana[5] says, these are

---

5 Dana, D (2020). *Polyvagal Exercises for Safety and Connection.* WW Norton & Company.

'anchors' or 'glimmers' – to soothe or stimulate ourselves, to calm or shift blocked energy and restore us to equilibrium, thereby reducing the triggers that would previously leave us craving a drink.

Anchors

These are resources we use to calm us down and soothe us if we find ourselves in the Sympathetic State of high arousal.

By looking around our environment we can identify resources – places and things that remind us of rest and safety – which act as a cue for our bodies to relax. What gives you the 'ahhhh', and makes you exhale and your shoulders drop? Perhaps it's your bed or a favourite chair where the sun hits it at 3pm and the light is just right. Maybe it's a soft blanket, essential oils or a favourite mug that feels at home in the palms of your hands, or it could be hugging a family member or a pet. If you can't go there immediately, sitting and breathing and calling them to mind can have a similar soothing effect on the mind and body, which can calm you down if you are stressed or anxious.

Glimmers

These are resources to bring us up, excite, connect and enliven us when we are in a Dorsal Vagal State of low arousal.

Sometimes, we may also need to pep ourselves up if we feel a bit stuck and flat. To do this, we need to activate the Ventral Vagal portion of our Autonomic Nervous System to connect and/or experience awe and wonder, happiness and excitement. What gives you a buzz or makes the hairs rise at the back of your neck with a shiver of excitement? Maybe switching on fairy lights or dancing to banging house music helps to enliven you and release pent-up stuff. Or it could be wild swimming, splashing your face with cold water or using a stimulating smell like eucalyptus, laughing with a friend or having a pillow fight.

Each person's menu will be different. Building these resources is about being curious, experimenting and seeing what feels good. Gradually we get better at reading the intel that comes through from our senses and nervous systems, earlier. When we learn to identify triggers and know what we need sooner, we can meet our needs more quickly as we grow in capacity and resilience.

Take a somatic break

Set your alarm five times during the day to take a two-minute somatic break from your surroundings. ('Somatic' means of the body, and a somatic break means switching off the mind and coming into the body.) Stare into space, close your eyes and focus on your breath, or rub the fingers of one hand against the palm and fingers of another hand – or lie down! Notice how you feel afterwards.

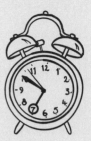

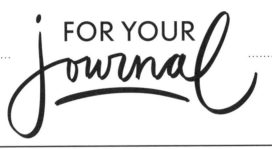

FOR YOUR Journal

What are my favourite spots in the house, park or natural world?
Where do I feel safe? Who do I feel safe with?
Where am I most relaxed?
What lights me up? What do I find beautiful?
What activates me into high arousal (makes me stressed)?

What activates me into low arousal (makes me want to hide away)?
What music excites me?
What music soothes me?

Because I was sober, this week I . . .

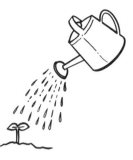

WEEK 7 :
FOSTERING POSITIVE GROWTH
Hope

'Hope is the thing with feathers -
That perches in the soul - And sings the tune
without the words - And never stops - at all.'
EMILY DICKINSON

Hope is believing that things are possible: it's a tiny spark in the darkness, a comforting thought that hard times will pass. When we embody the restorative energy of spring, we hope for the future, hope that we can sustain our sober journey, hope that things will get easier and that we can feel better. Our hope is fed by seeing tiny shoots of possibilities like the first daffs or crocuses in the snow. When we are hopeful, it's a bit like borrowing energy - hope keeps us going when our personal resources are depleted.

We need a big dose of hope and lots of motivation and support in the early days of sobriety. Sometimes, we can find hope within ourselves and sometimes we need to look outside for inspiration. We can look for evidence in people we find aspirational to keep that spark of hope going. It's the idea that if they can do it, maybe I can.

Hope is not about sitting around and dreaming; it's using the impulse of possibility to act. It helps us to remain focused on our goals and motivates us to keep working toward them. Although your own recipe for hope will come from your own needs and experience, experts say the cultivation of hope can be crystalized into three ways of thinking[6].

Let's explore how we can use these to boost our feelings of hopefulness in achieving an alcohol-free life:

1. Goals thinking – the clear visualization of goals important to us
   In sobriety, this means making the decision to be alcohol-free and knowing our reasons for this, perhaps, improved health, wealth and happiness, our kids, peace of mind, etc. If we can visualize the reality that this dream might just be possible, we can take the first step.

2. Pathways thinking – the ability to problem-solve to identify and develop specific strategies to reach those goals
   Joining a sober group, reading quit lit and learning how to deal with triggers are all examples of pathway thinking – the options you generate to help you keep going.

3. Agency thinking – the ability to initiate and sustain the motivation for using those strategies.

We need the push, the impetus to change – that bad hangover – the reason to do something different. We also need to believe that sober life might just be better and that it may be possible. We then need to keep motivated with connection and rewards – essentially, we need the sober toolkit and strategies in this book or whichever framework we find works.

---

6 Snyder, CR and Lopez, SJ (2002) *Handbook of Positive Psychology*. Oxford University Press..

Here are some suggestions of 'hope practices' to help you super-charge your hope mojo:

- Make your new habits instantly satisfying with Treat Friday. We invite you to treat/ reward yourself for every sober week. We reclaim Friday nights to do with as we please and no longer feel the FOMO (Fear of Missing Out). Treats can involve delicious food, box sets, cinema dates, bubble baths or using those calories we wasted on alcohol on something sweet instead.

- Make your sobriety socially rewarding by connecting with a sober group. You can be motivated by more people further down the line and meet new connections to cheer you on.

- Create a Pinterest or mood board and collate sober celebs you admire to help you learn by example. There are so many more of them out there than you might think

- Start with a challenge (such as Dry January) or have a day counter or a marble jar.

- Know that you don't have to re-start from day one after a slip, if it demotivates you (e.g. Kate is 5½ years sober at the time of writing but is 8 years, 7 months on the sober path).

- Tell yourself, 'I am a happy sober person', each day or, if that is a push, 'At least I didn't drink', or 'What are the lessons here?'

- Mark a calendar or stick gold stars in a wellbeing journal and celebrate milestones with special sober treats. These build motivation by satisfying the dopamine response in your brain, which looks for rewards, and also build sober muscle in your brain.

- Be a good news collector – collect positive stories to counteract the misery of the 24-hour news cycle bias. Also, do regular news fasts to protect your spirit. Switch off when you need to.

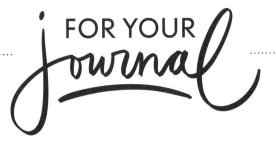
FOR YOUR
Journal

What is my recipe for hope?
What are the specific ingredients?
How can I add them into my day?
What makes me feel hopeful about alcohol-free living?

Who are my sober heroes and she-roes?
What evidence can I gather that I am capable of change?
Who inspires me?
How can I celebrate another day/week/month sober?

How do I feel about hope?
Do I feel hopeful? If yes, how can I build and share that?
If no, what needs to change? What are the things
blocking me from feeling hopeful?

How can I celebrate another challenge sober?

Because I was sober, this week I . . .

WEEK 8 :
EMOTIONAL TOOLKIT
Understanding the Hunger trigger

'An empty stomach is not a good political adviser.'
ALBERT EINSTEIN

One of the best-known sober acronyms is HALT, which stands for the triggers Hungry, Angry, Lonely, Tired, and this week we are looking at hunger. So many of us have dealt with poor body image and complicated relationships with food and dieting. The term 'drunkorexia' was invented to describe the habit of saving up calories for alcohol instead of food, and we can certainly resonate with that. Our bodies and minds need healthy fuel to be well, and lack of good nourishment can be devastating to our bodies and mental health. Many of us are running on empty tanks in many ways.

Spring is often a time associated with cleanses, juice fasts and diets but this may not be a good idea in your first sober spring, with hunger figuring as a major alcohol trigger. Eating regular snacks throughout the day, such as almonds, walnuts or fruit, has been proven to reduce cravings. This intentional focus on fuel through nutrition doesn't come easily for many of us perpetual dieters. The good news is that we can start to bring our diets into a greater balance. With calories freed up from quitting alcohol we can incorporate healthy fats, such as avocados and salmon, and other nourishing foods into our diets, which we may have been denying ourselves when counting calories.

When we stop drinking, it's common to experience sugar cravings and fluctuating blood sugar levels. If sweet treats help in the short-term then that is a win. It's important to focus on the one thing: don't try to detox, lose half a stone, crack sugar and quit alcohol all at the same time as its likely you will stumble. For sustainable wellbeing long term, we need to pace ourselves and, nature being our friend, if we choose things that can be grown or nourished from the earth rather than created in a factory, that's a good place to start healthy eating.

Hunger, of course, has emotional and psychological elements too. The Buddhist metaphor of The Hungry Ghosts has been used by psychologists Tara Brach and Dr Gabor Mate to illustrate the idea of the insatiable desire for more of a substance to make us feel better, fill emotional holes or alleviate suffering. When we stop drinking, we often become aware of uncomfortable feelings or stresses that the alcohol may have been masking, and so we need to start meeting those needs in healthy ways. The good news is that with the support of sober communities and with our growing sober toolkits, we get better and better at meeting our needs in positive ways rather than reaching for the bottle for the temporary (and counterproductive) fix.

Have fun by creating your own acronym of triggers. You can use it as a visual reminder when you are experiencing one.

KATE'S: HARIBO
Hungry • Angry • Resentful • Irritated • Bored • Overwhelmed

Mandy's: STOP
Stressed • Tired • Overwhelmed • Premenstrual

Neurotransmitter hack: dopamine – the rewarder

Alcohol or any addictive behaviour hits hard on the dopamine loop in the brain. In ancient times, the dopamine reward part of the habit loop was needed for our survival. How did it work? Seeing an animal was the CUE, which triggered the CRAVING to have the pleasure of feeling full. The RESPONSE was to hunt and kill the animal and the REWARD was to eat it, feel full and get the dopamine high. This was a sensible survival loop but, in the case of alcohol, it is being hijacked by an addictive chemical drug.

As we explained earlier in spring, alcohol depletes our own resources of dopamine so we become dependent on it. We also become tolerant to it, meaning it doesn't work as well in the same quantity and so we need more and more of it to get the rush. The dependence becomes greater and greater until we are in such a pleasure-deficient state, we find it hard to enjoy other activities that do not involve alcohol.

There are many ways to get healthy hits of dopamine and variety is the spice of life. In this sense, being sober is a lifetime of finding new ways of getting rewards so we don't get bored or dependent on something else. Pretty fun exploration!

Here are some natural ways to boost dopamine:

BRAIN FOOD

Foods thought to boost dopamine include:

- Chicken
- Cottage cheese
- Eggs
- Pork/turkey/duck
- Walnuts
- Oats
- Milk and yogurt

BODY FOOD

- Deep breathing
- Weightlifting
- Alternating nostril deep breaths

SOUL FOOD

- Celebrate your wins – small and big
- Tidy and clean
- Cross things off a 'to do' list
- Complete a task/ race/book/project
- Watch tv and films (especially 'high-reward' programmes such as makeover shows)
- Play games

FOR YOUR *Journal*

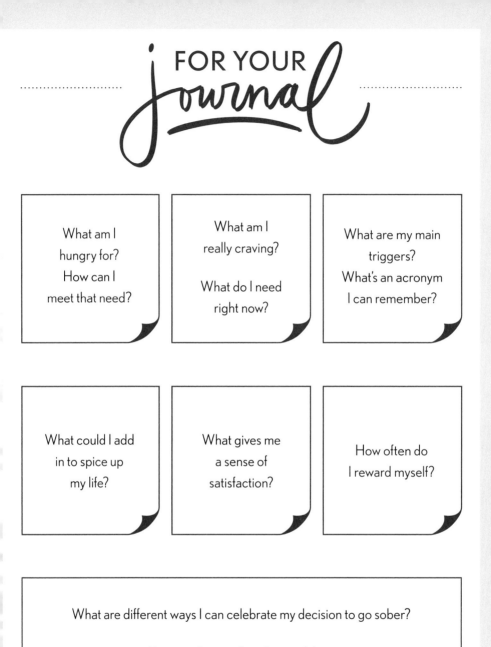

What am I
hungry for?
How can I
meet that need?

What am I
really craving?

What do I need
right now?

What are my main
triggers?
What's an acronym
I can remember?

What could I add
in to spice up
my life?

What gives me
a sense of
satisfaction?

How often do
I reward myself?

What are different ways I can celebrate my decision to go sober?

Because I was sober, this week I . . .

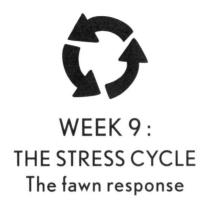

WEEK 9 :
THE STRESS CYCLE
The fawn response

*'When you say "Yes" to others, make sure you
are not saying "No" to yourself.'*
PAOLO COELHO

In our sober spring we can feel a bit like Bambi stuck in headlights, adjusting to new ways of being without alcohol. When we stop drinking and begin the sober journey, emotions, patterns and behaviours can come to the surface and we must be gentle with our fledgling springtime sober selves. This week we touch on something that has been talked about on sober forums for years among women, and often feels just part of what we do – the fawn response.

Fawning is more commonly known as people-pleasing. Perhaps you recognize that chameleon-like tendency of trying to fit in – it can be a strength, but can also come at a high price. We find the following definition of this behaviour from healthline.com to be the most succinct, 'Fawn types seek safety by merging with the wishes, needs and demands of others. They act as if they unconsciously believe that the price of admission to any relationship is the forfeiture of all their needs, rights, preferences and boundaries.'

When we learnt about the fawn response a lightbulb went on for both of us. Even naming it gave us agency to begin to change. We began to understand that our stress, resentment and drinking was connected with a survival technique, telling us it is better to say yes than to risk saying no and being rejected by the clan. When we realized this, we could begin to say no, learn tools to self-soothe, and ask better questions about our behaviour by legitimizing our own wants and needs.

Stress is your body's way of responding to any kind of demand or threat. As we mentioned in Week 5, when you sense danger, the body's defences kick into high gear in a rapid, automatic process known as 'fight or flight' or one of the other lesser-known stress responses, 'freeze or fawn.' Fawning, as discussed in Peter Walker's brilliant book *Complex PTSD: From Surviving To Thriving*, is a freeze response, often developed as a result of prolonged stress as a child.

For many years, there has been enormous stigma around addiction and problematic use of alcohol. It is seen as deviant, weak-willed and a moral failing, but if we reframe it as a response to trauma and stress, we can better understand it. We can have layers of trauma – childhood trauma, shock trauma or simply the trauma of overwhelm. As best-selling author Ann Dowsett Johnston writes, 'Alcohol has been used as the steroid that has enabled women to continue doing the heavy lifting of life.'

We cannot look after anyone if we are depleted and always in survival mode. So, if you have a tendency to people-please, know that you are not alone. But also know that the cost of being 'convenient' is often a feeling of profound separation, and despite our best efforts to connect we are at risk of parental burnout, work burnout and turning to alcohol to dial down the pressure.

Getting skillful at living with intention and putting yourself in the picture starts with knowing where you start and others end. It begins with saying no, with advocating for your needs and with the understanding that such actions aren't selfish but are imperative to your wellbeing. For some of us, this need to self-sacrifice for others' needs – even if they don't ask for it – can feel like an addictive behaviour in itself, which means it is damaging to healthy relationships.

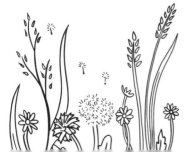

If, like us, you have struggled with setting boundaries and a tendency to people-please, it can help to gather some handy phrases to use:

"I need time to think about it, I will come back to you."

"I changed my mind." (No need for an explanation)

"I don't want to." (No need for an explanation)

"Sorry, I can't come." (No need for an explanation)

We delve further into boundaries in Summer, Week 6.

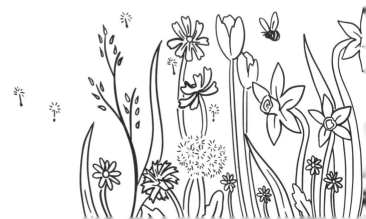

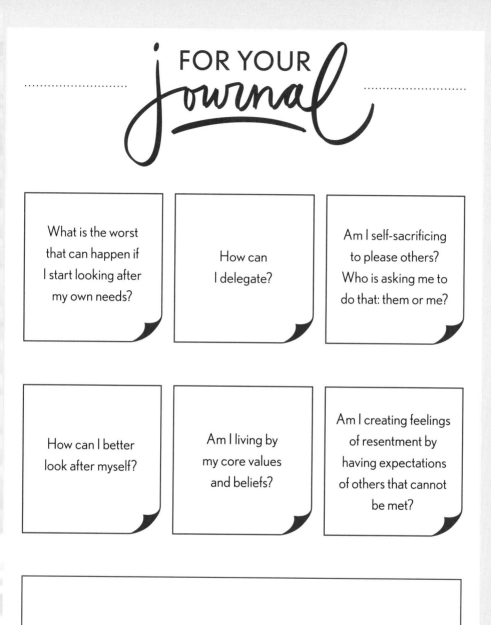

FOR YOUR journal

What is the worst that can happen if I start looking after my own needs?

How can I delegate?

Am I self-sacrificing to please others? Who is asking me to do that: them or me?

How can I better look after myself?

Am I living by my core values and beliefs?

Am I creating feelings of resentment by having expectations of others that cannot be met?

Because I was sober, this week I . . .

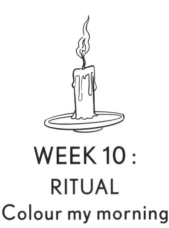

WEEK 10 :
RITUAL
Colour my morning

'The secret of your success is hidden in your daily routine.'
JOHN MAXWELL

Mornings are magical! Starting our day positively, with ourselves squarely in the centre, is one of the most powerful things we can do in our lives and in our sober journeys. Get up earlier than the kids/puppy/partner and take a delicious moment to breathe in the morning air. What better way to start the day than to sip a cuppa, wriggle your toes, congratulate yourself for another sober day and notice the sheer miracle that is each morning?

Every morning we have a chance to start again with a blank sheet and to set an intention for another sober day. All this instead of crawling out of bed with a hangover, looking in the mirror at bloodshot eyes, every noise making you wince as you juggle packed lunches or a commute with your arsenal of mints, shades and chewing gum, feeling that creeping regret that you did it again.

It's important to develop a morning routine that also works at weekends if need be. Sunlight, taking a deep breath, stretching, aligning your spine, adjusting your eyes, a leisurely coffee and becoming reacquainted with a different rhythm that suits a more restful non-work day sounds like a plan to us!

We can also carve out this space the night before by a little planning and prepping. Getting the school uniforms and running gear ready and sorting the packed lunches will create calm that you'll find you come to cherish and is so worth the effort. Claiming moments of stillness before the world wakes up is a bit like spring cleaning your time. Out with the old and in with the new!

By bossing our environments and the things we can control through routines and resources we can help avoid the stress building during the day. If we start frazzled, and add layers of stress throughout the day, we are more likely to hit the wine at 5pm. We can't always control all the stress of the day, but we can control the early bit before we see all the other feckers, at least most of the time.

Your morning routine doesn't always have to be exactly the same. If you want, you can mix it up using a colour chart like this:

	Monday	Tuesday	Wednesday	Thursday	Friday	Saturday	Sunday
Week 1	RED	BLUE	RED	GOLD	GREEN	GOLD	BLUE
Week 2	BLUE	GOLD	GOLD	BLUE	RED	RED	GREEN

Red routine: a 20-minute workout; hot shower; connect with friends.

Blue routine: meditate; stretch; soak in the bath; listen to favourite songs.

Gold routine: wear something you love; finish three important tasks, write a card to someone you love.

Green routine: get outside in nature; eat veggies all day, walk barefoot on grass; do a 10-minute workout.

By creating a chart like this, you make it easy on yourself (no indecision paralysis) while also holding yourself accountable (you've written it down so are more likely to follow and stick to it). Win-win!

WARNING Beware of any inner voice that tells you that you 'should' wake up at 5am to be more effective. Your morning requirements will change according to fluctuating energy levels, the stage of your cycle and your mood. Your routine is there to help, not be another stress. If you have poor sleep, then sleeping when you can will often be the most important thing you can do.

When you are in your inner spring you might be all over an early morning run, but if you're ovulating that may be the worst thing for you. You may have finally got your child to sleep by five and need to crash. Intentional living for good days and bad days to allow slack and self-compassion is the aim, rather than a military regime.

The most important message is that mornings are magical if you can make them. For us, sunrise beats sunset every time. Planning the night before is a gift and getting up an hour before the school run will help everyone. It's about manageable steps, so play with this to find what works for you and yours.

FOR YOUR *journal*

How can I create a morning routine?

What do I love about the morning?

How can I engage my senses in the morning?

What do I need in order to take time for myself?

Where is my starting point and where would I like to get to?

Can I play with going to bed earlier and getting up earlier? What's my energy like today?

Because I was sober, this week I . . .

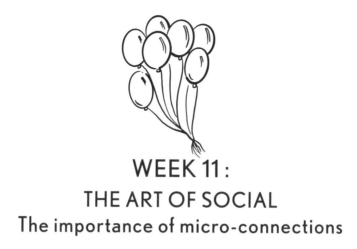

WEEK 11 :
THE ART OF SOCIAL
The importance of micro-connections

'We are hardwired to connect with others, it's what gives purpose and meaning to our lives and without it there is suffering.'
BRENÉ BROWN

Connection with others is a big issue when we get sober because we often see socializing through the narrow lens of parties, pubs or dinner parties. We worry that we won't be fun to be with and we'll never have fun again.

Slam on the brake right now – we need a reframe here! Being social does not have to mean sitting in a pub (yawn) or partying till dawn (eeeek), although it can be doing those things sober if you like. But it can also mean lunch with a friend or taking a yoga class. It can even mean having a chat with a shop worker, neighbour or delivery driver. In other words, getting our social needs met can be a combination of things including 'micro-connections'.

Micro-connections are like the tiny seedlings of connection – those small routine interactions throughout the day that we may not even be aware of, like a laugh with another dog owner or an authentic chat with another mum at the school gates, or even that glint of respect you can have when you catch someone's eye wearing a killer outfit. These little moments of connection peppered throughout the day can boost our feelings of positivity, connection and wellbeing.

In 2014, Essex University published research into the 'surprising power of weak ties',[7] which illustrated that micro-connections play a significant role in our wellbeing. Universities in Canada, the US and Turkey have also researched micro-connections and found that many people recalled a boost in mood when reaching out to others such as homeless people, shop workers, tradespeople, taxi drivers, and fellow hikers, campers or dog-walkers. During the pandemic teachers reported how missing short conversations outside of class time – in hallways, in the lunch line, at the door on the way into or out of school – impacted their day negatively.

It's often said that alcohol is a great leveller but that's because everyone gets boring after a bottle of wine. It is important to dispel the myth that alcohol makes social connection better. How can you have authentic connection with people when everyone has imbibed a mind-altering substance?

When we nurture small moments of connection in our everyday lives, we are less likely to feel like we are missing them and our brains collect evidence that we are getting our social cup filled. It's so much more nourishing for us to find connection in groups we feel a sense of belonging with – the fellow dog-walkers in the spring mornings, runners, women in a yoga class or even commuters on the train – as we cultivate our art of sober connection. We want no hangovers, no regrets and true connections – no matter how small.

A few years ago, I started an evening reflective practice to note my happiest moment in the day. I was surprised to find that even if I had bought something or treated myself to a facial, the moments that stood out were the micro-connections. A random, authentic chat with a school dad in the park or a shared laugh with an old lady in the supermarket, these were the happy hits that stuck. KATE

---

7 Sandstrom, GM & Dunn, EW (2014). *Social Interactions and Well-Being: The Surprising Power of Weak Ties*. Available at: pubmed.ncbi.nlm.nih.gov/24769739

I like to include these micro-connections in my gratitude practice, or 'happy hits' as I like to call them. I take a mental note – I am so glad I got to witness those cool socks, or see that guy's epic hairdo, I loved seeing that baby laugh or that chat with the bus driver. I do have to push myself to do this though, as I tend to become quite insular in my connections and I can definitely feel the difference when I connect with the world around me. MANDY

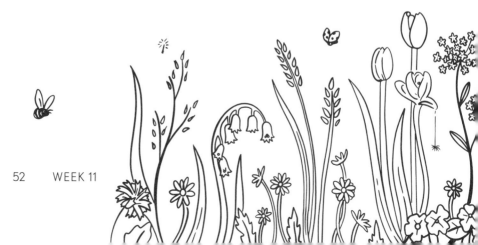

FOR YOUR *Journal*

Who are the micro-connections in my local neighbourhood?

What little random connections have I made today?

How can I engage a little more with people in my routine daily comings and goings?

What were my happiest moments today?

How connected do I feel to my local community? How can I build on that?

What stops me from connecting with people I don't know very well?

Would it be possible for me to slow down in order to join a class and arrive early enough to connect with other participants?

How do I feel after a nice chat with someone?

What can I do to dispel the myths I have about alcohol and socializing?

Because I was sober, this week I . . .

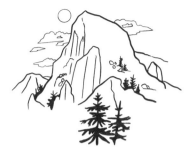

WEEK 12 :
THE SCHOOL OF LIFE
Going goddess on sobriety

'The inspiration you seek is already with you.
Be silent and listen.'
RUMI

As women, we ignite the power of the spring Goddess energy to carve out our own paths in sobriety. We rejected the 12-step sobriety programmes and refused to label ourselves as alcoholics, or accept we were powerless and had to live in a state of deprivation because we had a disease and couldn't do something 'ordinary' people could do. For much of our lives as women we have been competing in a patriarchal society, undoing the structures that make us feel 'less than', powerless or ashamed of ourselves, critical of our bodies and locked into gender-based roles of putting ourselves last. We weren't going to let another patriarchal model of recovery or alcohol dictate the story. We CHOSE sobriety as an empowered choice, as empowered women.

For many of us on sober forums, this journey had to be joyous; we needed to feel that we would gain more than we would lose by changing our habits and kicking booze to the curb, because quite frankly if it ain't got some sparkle we ain't signing up. Traditional models of recovery did not answer our needs in terms of being gender-appropriate or trauma-informed (though we are very grateful for those traditional models and recognize how much they have helped others). But necessity, as they say, is the mother of invention, so these two mamas got busy rewriting the rulebook!

We needed to feel positive, empowered, excited, hopeful. We wanted to feel better, make good friends, and have lives full of adventure and meaning. Sounds like a stretch? It honestly isn't. This is the possibility of new beginnings and of calling time on something that no longer serves you in order to rewrite your story.

Authentically engaging with our own individual processes of recovery rather than following others' rules was not always straightforward. At times we were confused and had periods of profound questioning. We also went back and forth to drinking (not that we wish that dance with the moderation hell on anyone) but we were searching for a model that felt true and authentic to make it stick. We felt as if we had lost ourselves in an entangled emotional relationship with alcohol that felt at times like an unbreakable bond. As our understanding grew, we could identify with a grey area of problematic drinking – or to put it another way, we were on the spectrum of alcohol addiction. To us, this looked like:

- Sometimes we drank too much
- Occasionally we binged to a dangerous level
- Often, we drank what would have seemed an 'ordinary' amount but it always left us filled with dread
- It impacted our mental wellbeing
- We held incredible shame about it
- We could start and stop without needing medical detox

When we were drinking, we felt profoundly disconnected from ourselves and when we stopped, we could finally listen in and look after ourselves and ask what we really needed. It's SO badass to be sober because we are intentionally asserting a boundary, choosing to be alcohol-free.

The conversation about 'grey-area drinking' resonates with many who do not identify with stereotypes of end-stage addiction. We want to feel better but are lacking the practical tools to manage stress. We lack adequate support and we are bombarded with BS about how 'mummy wine time' is all we need and deserve. We know that alcohol has a hold on us, we are worried about it, we have been trying to moderate and alcohol takes up A LOT of brain space. Make no mistake, going alcohol-free is the best solution for a grey-area drinker, as there is an addiction there, but we are not yet at that end stage (thank goodness) where medical intervention is needed in order to stop.

We believe that this decision to become free from alcohol is about reclaiming our own power and evolving better as badass sober females who are well and present, standing in our own authority to honour our pivotal role in our worlds and families. By living with intention, we choose to be alcohol-free because we will no longer harm ourselves or outsource our power to a bottle. We will focus on what's right about us and undo what, for many of us, has been a lifetime of self-harm, self-hate and self-abandonment. We will live in line with our bodies, needs and wants, and respect ourselves with boundaries as we actively create lives we love.

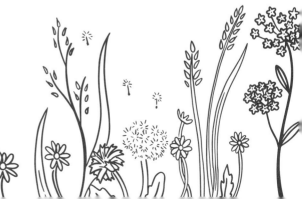

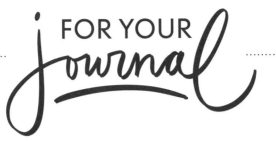

FOR YOUR *journal*

How would I like to claim my awesome decision to be alcohol-free?

What would I like to say to people about this awesome choice?

What does doing it my way look like?

What are the reasons that brought me to read this book?

How can I find ways to be supported emotionally,
mentally and physically?

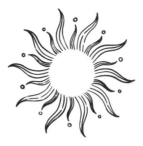

WEEK 13 :
TOOLS FOR GREATER REFLECTION
Self-care

*'Give yourself the same care and attention that
you give to others and watch yourself bloom.'*
ASHITA KUNJADIA

Developing your bespoke self-care practices is fundamental for your sobriety. So many of us spend our lives believing that self-care is selfish. Are you negating your own needs a) to keep the peace, b) because that's what you think you should do, or c) because you don't think you deserve time for you?

Both of us have had periods of burnout in our lives. Both of us were brought to our knees with regards to our self-worth, self-love and self-management with poor mental health and, for both of us, what consistently made these things worse was alcohol. As previously mentioned, Kate's sober mantra is, 'Sobriety is my fundamental act of self-care, which informs all others.' When we have gone back to drinking in the past, that self-care diminishes.

Self-care is so much more than treats and bubble baths. It is the toolkit and scaffold with which we build resilience and capacity. It is about self-leadership and cultivating a relationship with ourselves where we have our back. For each season, we are including some ideas for further enquiry to boost your journey, which will, in turn, impact your self-esteem and confidence further, strengthening your ability to meet your needs and reach your goals.

FOR SPRING WHY NOT:

- Stimulate your brain with new knowledge
- Start a new hobby
- Try something you find challenging
- Make time for documentaries and/or factual books to feed your curiosity
- Put in boundaries around work and take breaks
- Look into your money management – make a commitment to a budget to enable future security and fun
- Create space for play, be it in arts, crafts, puzzles, games or sports
- Invest in some lovely moisturizer, face packs, scrubs and bath balls to create yourself a spa ritual
- Sleep more
- Read more
- Get out in nature more
- Turn your phone off more

Spring is a brilliant time to look at your environment through a self-care lens, get rid of the old and make room for the new. We can do some serious decluttering of mind, body and soul at this time of year. So why not allow some gentle enquiry around the things you DO, HAVE and ARE in your life? Ask yourself:

Is this useful? Do I need it? Does it make me happy?

If you answered no to two or more of those questions, ask yourself:

Can I get rid of this to make space?

AREAS OF ENQUIRY MAY BE:

- Your knicker and sock drawer – we know you know . . .
- Your food cupboards
- Your clothes
- The things you say about yourself
- Your environment – professionally and personally
- Your shame

SPRING EQUINOX
Ritual and reflection

*'Spring drew on . . . and a greenness grew over those brown beds,
which, freshening daily, suggested the thought that hope traversed
them at night and left each morning brighter traces of her steps.'*
CHARLOTTE BRONTË

The word equinox comes from the Latin words for 'equal night' – *aequus* (equal) and *nox* (night). On the equinox, the length of day and night is nearly equal in all parts of the world.

The Spring Equinox sees a time of rebirth in nature, with flowers coming out and baby animals being born, and with it comes hope and possibility. We are beginning to look outward, spending more time outdoors as we move energetically from the introversion of the winter months to greater activity and extroversion, like a butterfly ready to burst from its chrysalis.

Full of potent energy, we turn our faces to the sun in the promise of lighter days with the dark, cold days of winter receding behind us. It's a time of huge celebration, with many sacred holidays in the Northern Hemisphere such as Easter (Eostre) and Mayday (Beltane) focused on fertility and rebirth – beautifully nourishing for the RESTORE part of the R4 BALANCE method – and it's hard not to feel excited to see the new signs of life and welcome that extra vitamin D.

Despite its inherent positivity, however, this first transition point can be challenging. In our first sober year, we both noticed a pattern emerging in the form of a low point or lull every three months or so. We realized that these transition points wove themselves through the changing cycles of our sobriety as well as having inherent shifts around the physical seasons. During the first cycle of sobriety, this three-monthly low ebb was disconcerting – we certainly wondered where our sober mojo had gone and were relieved when it picked up again after a week or so.

Our focus on the restorative nature of spring, with growth and preparation for the next season, fortifies us as we move through the year. The equinox provides that opportunity to pause and integrate the learning of the season. When we pause, we can honour the delicate balance of 'all.the.things': ourselves, our needs, the environment, our energy levels. We draw breath and give thanks before we move on to the next stage, activity or project, acknowledging our efforts and progress, which in turn grows our self-esteem. So, let's take a minute to consciously build this in at the global transitions of equinox and respect smaller or more personal transitions too.

FOR YOUR Journal

How is my experience of springtime energy?
How do I feel about being alcohol-free as I head into warmer days?
What dreams do I want to have take root and grow in my life?
What were my wins?
What challenges did I overcome?
What am I proud of?
How will I reward myself?
What am I ready to let go of?
What do I need to shed in order for new life to grow?
If I secretly knew the answer – what would it be?
Because I was sober, this week I . . .

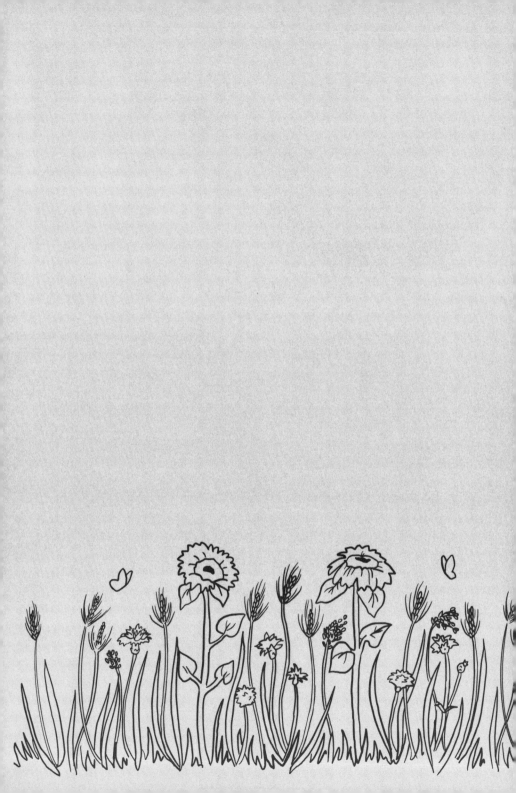

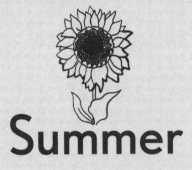

Summer

'Rest is not idleness, and to lie sometimes on the grass
under trees on a summer's day, listening to the murmur
of the water, or watching the clouds float across the
sky, is by no means a waste of time.'
JOHN LUBBOCK

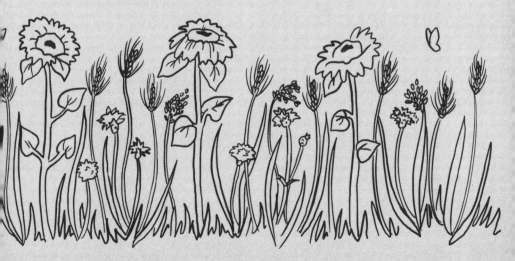

HARNESSING THE POWER OF
THE GIFTS OF SUMMER TO REIGNITE

As we head into summer, our sobriety has matured slightly and we can use the energy of the season to reignite our passion for hobbies, creative practices and all that was left by the wayside when booze danced centre stage. The warmth and light of summer can also fortify us for deeper work and the coming darker months. We are entering a new cycle with our sobriety. It's connected to the next stage of the R4 Balance Method – REIGNITE – where we embrace our sober choice and create action to change, while at the same time respecting the need to conserve what we have started. With this new territory comes some adjustment and a change of gear as we head into this sociable, energetic season with its gifts of light and warmth, increased sociability, outside activities and holidays.

We have had enough sober time to reap some benefits of sowing our sober seeds and intentions. We may enjoy improved sleep and energy levels, our moods may have levelled, and typically we are feeling more confident in our sober choice. However, summer can also be a cluster trigger with its association with high days, holidays and the pursuit of pleasure. But let's face it, hangovers in the heat are no cause for celebration. So, how do we enjoy the benefits of the fiery season, while avoiding its danger spots?

During each new cycle in our new habit we are challenged once again to adapt our sober toolkit to whatever the conditions. Just as you wouldn't wear a bikini in the rain, we need to choose the right tools for the job. During the period of school closure, aka the summer holidays, there is a tendency to run ourselves ragged, forget the early lessons of building our sober toolkit and self-care, and find ourselves triggered to drink again. We may be venturing out more, feeling more sociable with the summer's extrovert energy. We need to be aware that we also have to rest and rehydrate, and restock our toolkits, like packing picnic hampers for long days out. It's important to note the emergence of fading affect bias (that we forget how bad things were over time) and our vulnerability to seeing things through rose-tinted sunglasses, which makes rosé all day suddenly seem like a great idea.

In this section, we work with the heat and activity of summer and the idea of maintenance to explore how to set boundaries, manage our social life and cope with being sober in a busy world. This way we can look after ourselves and enjoy the sunshine, longer evenings and holidays happy, healthy and alcohol-free.

Return to this section whenever you feel like you have hit a plateau on your sober journey and you want to spark joy, get excited and reignite your sober passion. It will also help you find balance and conserve what you have built so far when summer's pace has left you depleted and/or overwhelmed and you need tools to help you put on the brakes and manage energetic and overwhelming times in your year.

REASONS TO BE CHEERFUL IN SUMMER

Ice creams, long evenings, the patio, sunshine, warmth, the seaside, flipflops, manicures, sunflowers, blue sky.

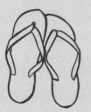
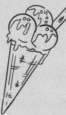
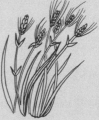

FOR YOUR JOURNAL

How do I want to feel this summer?

What matters to me the most this season?

When do I feel at my most happy/calm/joyful in summer?

What would I like to create or nurture in my life this season?

What elements make summer special for me?

What fears would I like to release this summer?

Because I was sober, this week I . . .

WEEK 1:
YOUR SEASONAL PLANNER

*'If you don't know where you are going,
you'll end up someplace else.'*
YOGI BERRA

Let's have a look at the overview of your summer. As with spring, we are designing our life map according to the natural features and lay of the land and planning our route to better prepare for our journey. With summer being a particularly busy time generally, and including the period of school closure, planning and taking things off the list can help us so much. So, let's reflect on holidays or extra family commitments coming up. What challenges did this season bring in the past? Is it particularly difficult to keep going on your sober journey when the sun shines? What fun things can you discover? What have you got to look forward to?

Fill in the simple planner to note your intentions for specific dates and some questions for deeper reflection to get your summer game plan on!

SUMMER
Planner

Month 1

Month 2

Month 3

Hobbies to try ....
....
....

Key dates

Possible Triggers

Strategy...
Movement ....
Self-care ....

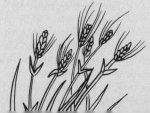

HOW TO USE YOUR PLANNER FOR SUMMER

Reigniting passion in your life is as much about saying yes as it is about saying no. A life you love sober is about widening your choices and trying out new things, but also knowing when to politely decline things. If this is your first sober summer, a four-day long festival might not be the one this year ... or maybe it is? Adjust your self-care to suit the summer warmth and energy. Do you feel like changing up your exercise? Have relaxing hot baths become cool showers in your life?

As with the other seasons, we challenge you to:

- Choose a social activity that you want to try alcohol-free
- Try a new alcohol-free drink
- Do a new hobby or activity that you have always wanted to try
- Say no to something you don't want to do
- Add in some movement

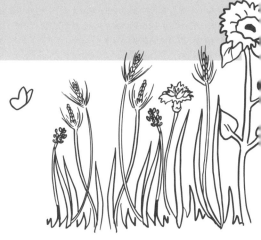

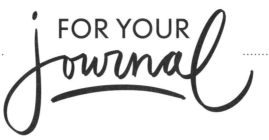

FOR YOUR
Journal

What associations do I have with these major dates coming up?
How confident on a scale of 1–10 do I feel about managing this
period alcohol-free?
Which activities do I want to opt out of this year?

What key dates have I identified that are important to me?
How do they normally relate to drinking alcohol? What new rituals can I introduce?
Are there certain dates I need to plan around because of alcohol?
What will I do?

What do I need to do to increase my confidence level by 1 point?
(Have a friend there, opt out, drive, journal more, get a coach?)
What might I do instead?
What might I drink instead?

What can I plan in instead?
Because I was sober, this week I . . .
What is your confidence level now out of 1-10? Hopefully it will have improved.
If not, go back and see if you can generate more options to encourage you.

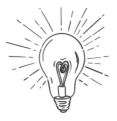

WEEK 2 :
SETTING YOUR INTENTION
Honesty

'Be yourself; everyone else is already taken.'
OSCAR WILDE

A beautiful and inevitable part of stopping using alcohol as a coping mechanism is that we get to see the rich beauty of our lives and the natural world surrounding us without booze goggles. This can also be confronting, however, as we are no longer numbing the edges or the hurts. It is ironic that we use alcohol in the pursuit of pleasure and in the avoidance of pain, and yet alcohol then both invites pain into our lives with its addictive nature and reduces our capacity to enjoy pleasure.

When we are caught up in the cycle of problematic drinking, we carry a lot of shame. This results in a belief that we don't have the right to advocate for ourselves because we are letting ourselves and others down. Frankly, we often don't have the capacity either. But knowing day in and day out that we are meeting our goal to stay alcohol-free will give us strength and confidence in ourselves. It allows us to become more honest with our kids, our partners and our friends about what we need, want and enjoy.

Over time, without the influence of alcohol, as you move past the initial discomfort, you get to sense your edges and the truth of how you experience your life, relationships and environment. This is actually the biggest gift anyone can receive, even if it doesn't feel like it at first. Once we can see clearly, we get to design our lives with honesty and intention.

We noticed ourselves becoming more honest and braver in this second cycle, more articulate when asking for what we needed and in advocating for ourselves. Perhaps we just got tired of things that were not really working. We became more honest in our conversations because there was nothing to hide behind, and we felt increasingly able to turn down invites to things we didn't feel like going to and speak up about things that p***ed us off. We were also able to articulate more clearly our needs because we understood them with greater clarity. People responded to us better because we were using our honesty calmly and consistently. In this way, our truth-telling was safer for those around us and gave them the opportunity and space to be truthful back.

The first step toward living authentically and honestly is to tell the truth to yourself about your relationship with alcohol. Only you know how bad it is or feels or was or felt. (Please also refer to the Resources section for the World Health Organization's breakdown of alcohol use disorder and next steps to get help.) So, when those summer vibes hit and it triggers noise from the Wine Witch or Beer Fiend that you weren't that bad or you can control your drinking, be really honest with yourself. Can you really? Do you really want to? How did that 'moderation' really work out? Alcohol doesn't change, so it will still have the same impact if you go back. You haven't come this far to only come this far.

Don't be afraid of the honest truth. The truth is, you are a valuable member of the human race and deserve your place and your voice. There is no rush, you can take your time. Much of the timeline in this book is metaphorical and you may have many, many months of spring, or you may feel like this only in your second summer. It's your journey.

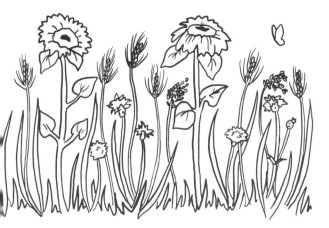

"We noticed ourselves becoming more honest
and braver in this second cycle, more articulate
in asking for what we needed and in
advocating for ourselves."

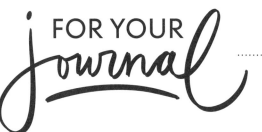

FOR YOUR Journal

Take an honest look at yourself and alcohol:

What are my early memories of alcohol?

What was the relationship with alcohol like in my family?

How old was when I started drinking alcohol?

Why did I drink? What need did it meet at the time?

Can I remember any significant moments when my relationship with alcohol changed to become problematic?

How has my sleep been impacted by alcohol?

How has my mental health been impacted by alcohol?

Do I/did I see alcohol as a treat? Why?

Was I honest? What did it tell me?
Have I accepted that alcohol is addictive? That alcohol dependency is a spectrum from mild, moderate to major? How hard is it for me to stop and stay stopped? Because I was sober, this week I . . .

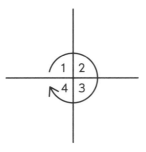

WEEK 3:
CYCLES AND SOBRIETY
Calling BS on the Cult of Youth
(It's OK not to go to the party)

'Wanton kittens make sober cats.'
OLD ENGLISH SAYING

Have you ever considered how ideas of aging and youth impact on how you drink? This strange 'kidult' mix of responsibility, proper jobs and mortgages while trying to continue the lifestyle we had when we were young and carefree is wreaking havoc on our bodies, minds and nervous systems. It's time to go home before we turn into pumpkins!

Somewhere in the heady mix of Converse trainers, stripy Boden T-shirts, skinny jeans and prosecco, we have lost sight of the fact that life does move forward and we can change with it. If we are to live intentionally and aligned with our natural rhythms, our lifestyles need to be evolving to match this inevitable aging process – and to honour it. We beat ourselves up for not doing everything and being everything to everyone and push ourselves constantly. In turn, we become even more depleted and dysregulated and more likely to turn to alcohol to soothe and relax us, which, as we know, dysregulates and depletes us further.

We are bombarded with images in the media of celebrities who are bossing the midlife but what we don't see is the whole team of people they have managing their diet, surgeries, diary, childcare, wardrobe etc., etc. It doesn't mean that you have to embrace nanny cardigans and never go to a festival again (unless that sounds dreamy) but what we are checking here is your energy levels and the reality for everyday women.

Summer is a trigger time for partying, kicking up our heels and being outside in the long evenings with the allure of civilized sun-downers – but perhaps now you have identified that you don't want to drink like you used to, otherwise why would you be reading this book? The hangovers are too costly, the anxiety rife, the sleepless nights awful. You have been aspiring to 'grow up' and drink 'like an adult' yet find yourself still bingeing like you did when you were 18, holding on to the notion that 'moderating' alcohol is the holy grail of adult drinking yet, in reality, you feel ashamed to be rolling out of the bar with your younger colleagues like it's Happy Hour circa 1999. Maybe everyone around you is the same, but they don't seem to care as much as you? It can be very challenging when we want to change but everyone else seems to want to stay the same.

Life is supposed to be a series of cycles. We grow and we learn, and we develop wisdom as we grow. We often get caught looking back and trying to emulate what has already been, rather than looking forward to where we are going and how we would like our future to be. Life isn't about holding on to the past, and it isn't about the destination (or maybe it is to you). For us, it's the journey, the experience of being informed by the past to live in the present and look forward to the future, all the while cherishing our health and living mindfully in the moment.

Life is a lot. We can get stuck sometimes with the impact of events like illness, bereavement, shock, trauma, lack of support – so many things. But drinking does not help any of these. Part of growing up is living through the stuff and finding ways to seek the support we need to deal authentically with life on life's terms. Aging is just one of those terms.

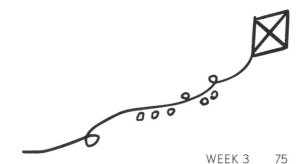

For us, motherhood was the catalyst that both accelerated our alcohol dependence and made us finally realize that something had to change. We were no longer only responsible for ourselves, yet we were behaving in irresponsible or dangerous ways when drunk and could ignore it no longer. No shame, no blame – this is what happened. The heightened stress, overwhelm and dysregulation led us to drinking more to dial down and unwind. Alongside the normalization of 'mummy wine time', this built up to the perfect storm. It was simply not sustainable.

Whether we are parents or not, the cycles of life keep turning and our bodies need extra care. We may be in the perimenopause, menopause or post-menopausal. Wherever we are in our cycles of life, we need to adapt to thrive and survive.

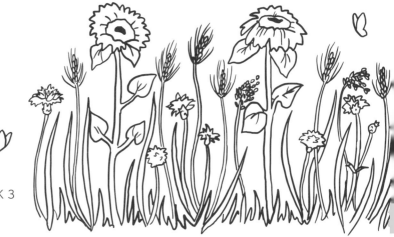

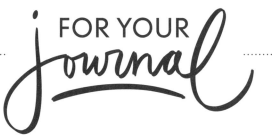

FOR YOUR *journal*

What is it about my life that makes me feel resentful, trapped or stuck?

What can I do to change the things that no longer serve me?

Do I have friends who have transitioned into being in their adult lives, and others who are still acting as they did in their late teens?

What are the values that are important for me to live by at this stage in my life?

What first step can I take in moving toward a life that suits my energy better?

Because I was sober, this week I . . .

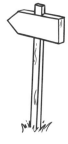

WEEK 4 :
CULTIVATING SOBER SPACE
Challenging our beliefs

'We construct our beliefs, mostly unconsciously, and thereafter they hold us captive.'
DAVE GRAY

'Alcohol helps me relax', 'People will think I'm boring', 'Drinking is sophisticated', 'It's what adults do', 'But what will I do at Christmas?', 'People will assume I have a problem.' . . . Do any of these beliefs sound familiar to you? We have great news for you – an alcohol-free life is the best kept secret! But first we need to do some myth-busting . . .

Because alcohol is what we call 'socially normative' we have all kinds of unconscious beliefs about how normal it is to drink and how abnormal it is not to. These drivers governing our habits and behaviour are our unconscious beliefs, which come from our family of origin, culture, our peers, advertising, films, TV and social media. So, we need to be reality detectives when we stop drinking, and challenge the messages we receive about alcohol.

We engage the emotional brain to help empower our habits. (Remember the elephant and rider? see page 23) . . . we must also undo the brainwashing that affects our emotional brain too. By really analysing the unconscious bias toward alcohol and challenging its truth for us, we can build sober muscle.

When we start to investigate these beliefs, challenge them and discount them with evidence – and see the marketing machine behind this – we take hold of a golden ticket to getting rid of the Wine Witch for good.

THREE STEPS TO WORK WITH UNCONSCIOUS BELIEFS

Let's take one of the many common myths around drinking: 'Alcohol helps me relax'.

1. Ask questions and challenge your perceptions

Ask yourself, am I sure it helps me to relax? Because being hungover all weekend certainly doesn't feel relaxing and, come to think of it, waking up at 4am makes me super anxious . . . Also, I never really relax at a party because I am always counting my drinks and watching the bottle. And what does it mean to relax anyway?

2. Seek facts and knowledge

Read books on the subject, listen to podcasts, know so much that you can't unknow it. Here are a couple of pertinent examples.

FACT: We know from science that alcohol is both a stimulant and a depressant – the first glass of wine may imitate the feeling of being relaxed but it's really an ineffective bandage for stress and anxiety because it makes you more stressed and anxious in the long run. So, it doesn't relax you at all.

FACT: Alcohol depletes your brain and your body of the ability to relax by itself so you become reliant on it, and then it stops working and you're just chasing not having withdrawal from it, which is not in any way relaxing.

3. Investigate what works instead and do it

What really relaxes me? What can I do that will help me more? Maybe take that bath, go to bed early, work on boundaries, remove a stressor from my life, go to the theatre, take a walk or go for a swim?

The reality of our drinking was not relaxing. It was falling over, feeling ashamed, waking up with our makeup still on, neglecting promises to friends and family, feeling irresponsible, having the same conversation over and over and never being fully present. Alcohol systematically took away more than it gave.

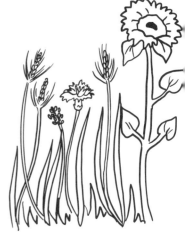

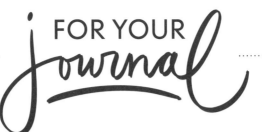

FOR YOUR journal

Take a look at some of the myths you may hold about alcohol, such as:

> Alcohol helps me relax
>
> I can't have fun without alcohol
>
> I can't connect with others without alcohol
>
> Alcohol makes me sophisticated
>
> Alcohol is a treat
>
> Drinking alcohol is part of romance
>
> It is empowering for a woman to drink
>
> Drinking is part of being a feminist
>
> I can't get through motherhood without alcohol

Now ask yourself:

> What is the story I tell myself about alcohol?
>
> What is my reality really like?
>
> What are the facts?
>
> What can I do instead?
>
> Because I was sober, this week I . .

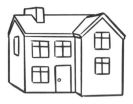

WEEK 5 :
BOSSING YOUR ENVIRONMENT
Let it be easy

'I will always choose a lazy person to do a difficult job because a lazy person will find an easy way to do it.'
BILL GATES

One of the key factors in successful habit change is making the new habit as easy as possible for ourselves. One of the reasons that this evidence-based nugget of wisdom eluded us for the first year of our sobriety was that we were focusing on trying really hard, and when you are trying really hard at something it can actually make it harder. If your approach to sobriety is gritting your teeth and saying to yourself, 'I won't drink, I won't drink, I won't drink', it's going to be a very long year.

Summer is nature's way of letting things be easy for a bit (then we had to go and invent the school holidays!). In nature, there is an abundance of food and the harsh days of winter are behind us. Nowadays, the summer days allow us to enjoy coffees outside in the morning, an ice cream in the park, long hazy evenings and easier school runs as we are not braced against the elements. The extra light boosts our vitamin D and serotonin levels and this extra energy is perfect to reignite our love for life and everything we can gain from our choice not to drink.

We are not making light of the effort that we put into changing our habits and our relationship with alcohol. It definitely takes work, but with a few tips and tools, some support and a bit of time under our belt it can feel a whole lot easier – and the good bits keep getting better!

OUR MENU FOR YOUR EASY SOBRIETY

Get clear on your 'why'

Identify some core values you have in the areas of family, health, mental health, money or greater productivity. Then link your decision to be sober to one of those values, for example: I am sober so I can have energy to enjoy time with my kids. Or 'I am sober to boss my yoga'.

Move

One of the reasons we use alcohol is to alleviate stress. Mindful movement to de-stress is essential to boost our neurotransmitters of dopamine and serotonin. If you can release the stress, you will find wine o'clock will pass. Swimming, a few minutes of yoga, self-massage in the bath or a walk may seem like nothing but they prompt your brain to recognize it's time to switch gear and relax.

Mealtimes

Eat earlier in the evening to curb booze cravings. Your blood sugar levels drop after a tiring day leaving you depleted and undernourished, which is a huge trigger. Food is usually less associated with alcohol in our minds the earlier it is in the day/evening and eating with the kids, or when you get home from work can break the routine and create a new alcohol-free ritual.

Get into nature

Connecting with nature soothes our nervous systems and a walk at the end of the day can help you dial down a booze trigger.

Hug and chat to people and pets

Soothe and connect with furry things and people and even hug yourself to boost oxytocin and make you feel loved and connected.

Practise self-compassion

If you stumble, don't beat yourself up. Reflect on what worked for you, what didn't and what you can do differently. We are all learning.

See yourself in partnership with the Universe

When we are trying to control all the things for all the people in all the areas of our lives, things feel like a grind. When you let it go, send it out to the Universe and focus on being well, things feel lighter.

Keep what works and leave the rest

Even in our own feelings we can get caught up in trying to always do the next thing. We forget what worked in the first place because we feel like we need to deepen the recovery. If colouring, having a bath and watching Netflix keep you sober, then that is enough.

FOR YOUR *journal*

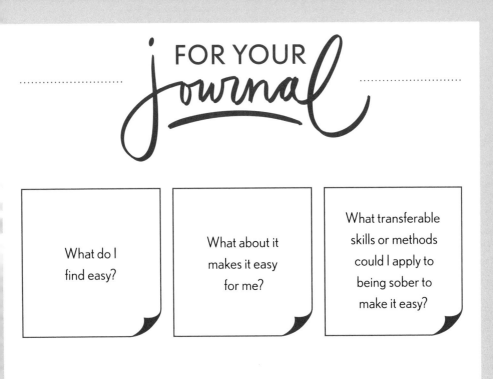

What do I find easy?

What about it makes it easy for me?

What transferable skills or methods could I apply to being sober to make it easy?

What times of the day is it easy to be sober? Why is that? What does that tell me about stress/my need for breaks and rest throughout the day?

In what situations do I find it easy to be sober?

How can I make it even 1% easier?

Because I was sober, this week I . . .

WEEK 6 :
RESEARCHING OUR RESOURCES
Boundaries

'When we fail to set boundaries and hold people accountable to them, we feel used and mistreated.'
BRENÉ BROWN

Boundaries are our guidelines to what is acceptable to us and essential to our mental health, wellbeing and sobriety. Boundaries can be external (those we have with other people) and internal (those we have with ourselves). Setting external and internal boundaries shows respect for others and for yourself. They are essential for maintaining healthy interdependent relationships that are neither enmeshed (no boundaries) nor detached (too many boundaries). When we have healthy boundaries, we feel safe, cared for and have trust in ourselves and others.

Summer can be a tricky time for boundaries because it's so often the time when our routines go a bit wonky. Just one example of this is the long summer school holidays that usually result in our kids going to bed later and getting up later, and mealtimes taking on a life of their own. And when routines go, so do the boundaries they help keep in place. We can insert the annual summer holiday here too, where normal rules don't apply and we can come home worse off than when we left because it feels acceptable to drink from noon.

In sobriety, boundaries are a key issue that people struggle with and after the early muscle power exercised during the first three months, this can become apparent.

On a deeper level, many of us coming into sobriety don't actually know what boundaries are. We are not people who ever had a boundary around alcohol intake – it was never 'just one'. You are reading this book probably because you identify with not having an off switch when it comes to alcohol. We believe that one of the most fundamental boundaries we ever created was saying no to alcohol. Then, all the other boundaries became much easier because we took this first step.

Those that have a tendency to develop a problematic relationship with alcohol often put others' needs first. Left unchecked and without suitable boundaries in place, this can lead to overwhelm and resentment. We can feel unheard, unloved and unseen and this feeds in to the cycle of drinking because we are fed the lie that alcohol is a treat we deserve to cope with difficult feelings. Alcohol then becomes something sacred – we build a boundary around 'me and my wine', we actually get left alone to rest if we're hungover – and none of this helps our mental and physical wellbeing in the long run.

DEFINING BOUNDARIES

....

Boundaries can be:

Physical You are entitled to your own personal space, privacy and safety.

Mental Your mind is your own. You get to decide what thoughts to think and what information you allow to come in. For instance, if watching the news upsets you, you can choose not to watch it.

Additionally, you do not have to share your thoughts, opinions or beliefs if you choose not to. You also do not have to listen to the thoughts, opinions or beliefs of others if you choose not to. You have the right to protect your own thought space.

Material You should have an expectation of privacy when it comes to your material possessions. For instance, you may keep a journal that you do not want your significant other to read. This is perfectly OK. Or you may not want to share with others how much money you make.

Emotional You have permission to experience emotional health and wellness. Emotional boundaries should be firmly rooted in the knowledge that you are responsible for your own feelings and that you are NOT responsible for the feelings of others. In other words, someone cannot make you feel a certain way. You choose your own emotional responses, just as they choose theirs.

Spiritual Spiritual boundaries promote your spiritual health and you are entitled to protect them. You may do this quietly and respectfully. There is no need to explain your spirituality to anyone else, nor is it appropriate to force your beliefs on someone who believes differently from you.

By the time most people get sober, the relationship they have with themselves is in a bit of a state – it certainly was for us. Rebuilding self-confidence and experiencing self-love is an ongoing process that takes time and practise. You start to rebuild the relationship you have with yourself by making the commitment to stay sober one day at a time. This could be the first conscious internal boundary you set with yourself. As you live up to this commitment with each passing day, you will feel more comfortable in your own skin and grow with confidence. We named this season REIGNITE in our R4 Balance Method because getting sober is the first step in powerful reclamation of everything you loved before your life got tarnished with booze. It is a flame that reignites in you the spark for life, the strength in your decisions and self-leadership in your life.

Doing this will enable you to set other boundaries with more clarity, such as boundaries about what you eat, how often you exercise, how you spend your money, what time you go to bed every night and what time you wake up every morning. Setting internal boundaries is a true practice of self-care and self-love. After years of using alcohol to blur the edges, this may seem foreign at first – but with time it will become second nature, we promise.

FOR YOUR *journal*

How can I respect my internal and external boundaries?

Are there any boundaries that are being compromised?

What's the one thing I could do to improve a boundary that feels vulnerable?

What will I gain from strengthening my boundaries?

How will working on my boundaries help my sobriety journey?

Because I was sober, this week I . . .

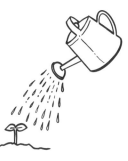

WEEK 7 :
FOSTERING POSITIVE GROWTH
Kindness

*'Three things in human life are important:
the first is to be kind; the second is to be kind;
and the third is to be kind.'*
HENRY JAMES

Summer is a naturally sociable time – we may chat to our neighbours more as we are out in our gardens again, we spend longer up and out because of the longer days, and we may linger by the school gates or in the park longer because we are not huddled and bracing ourselves against the cold. We might meet up with colleagues after work or do a group sport and hang out afterwards – things feel less like hard work for many of us. This natural tendency toward social interactions gives us the opportunity to observe and participate in kindness practices.

Kind actions and words are like a social glue that binds us together. Kind actions can shift a sh*tty mood. Kindness fosters our feelings of being connected, which lights up our mirror neurons in the brain. These brain connectors fire up both when we act and when we observe the same action performed by another. The neurons release serotonin and oxytocin and it feels gooooood as it mirrors what it sees as if the observer itself were doing the action. Scientists in Berkeley and Harvard discovered that the brains of people watching strangers being kind to each other lit up the same regions as when people were kind to them!

This can be a great time for extroverts who get energy from interaction in groups – all that kind energy will be flowing just great – you crack on dudes! For those of us who are prone to fitting in and people pleasing, we need extra TLC and tools around kindness – we need to remember to give it to ourselves first because we can get depleted and end up giving too much of ourselves to other people.

In the philosophical texts of yoga, kindness is known as 'ahimsa' or 'do no harm' ('a' – no, 'himsa' – harm). This applies to everything: being kind in all that we think, say and do. Kindness, however, needs to start with ourselves if we are to be successfully and actively kind to others. It's the old 'put on your own oxygen mask before helping others' analogy. It's interesting to look at alcohol through the lens of ahimsa. Alcohol does enormous harm to body and mind and so if we are to care about kindness, we can use this as a good reason to not imbibe a poisonous carcinogen. If we recall the times we have said mean things while under the influence – booze-fuelled late-night arguments, or the mornings we have woken up full of shame and beaten ourselves up because of the night before – we can see that removing alcohol from the mix is the kindest thing we can do for ourselves and for those we love.

For me, being a witness to kindness or participating in kindness helps me feel less isolated, which was a huge trigger for me. When I am part of a world and can see evidence of kindness it helps me feel hopeful, which in turn sparks the feelings of possibility. It's not surprising that so many people find being part of a sober community so rewarding (yay, dopamine!) because helping others helps us. MANDY

My own journey has been to reclaim kindness and non-harming toward myself.
I had a vicious inner critic and spent a good deal of my life cut off from my
feelings. Through yoga and working weekly with the principles of ahimsa
I have incorporated kindness into my life in a more balanced way. Seeing
random acts of kindness makes me cry! I often feel like they are divine.
One of the weirdest things I remember is what happened last year when I
made a cake for my neighbour whose husband had recently passed. When my
daughter and I delivered it, it turned out to be the neighbour's birthday and
none of her family had made a cake because they were all mourning. It was a
powerful moment for us both and strengthened our bond as neighbours. KATE

There are so many resources around kindness, so we encourage enquiry into a balanced approach to help you get the right recipe for you. Kindness to others can be practised consciously when you feel energized and have extra to give, and directed to yourself when you need it. The sunny (hopefully) summer season is an ideal time to bake a cake for a neighbour, pick up litter, rescue puppies – whatever lights you up.

If the last couple of years of the pandemic have taught us anything, it's how MUCH we need other people, and not just our nearest and dearest, but our wider community, our support networks – be it our hairdresser or the post-person. When in doubt, you can look for cues of kindness from others – watch a gardening or makeover show, sign up to positive news sites and kindness accounts on Instagram – it can all make a difference on a difficult day.

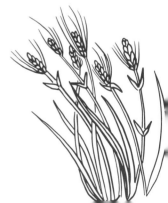

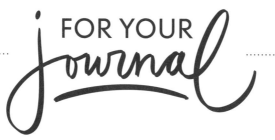
FOR YOUR *Journal*

What is the one thing I can do to be kind to myself today?
How can I rest?

Check my mood. What's the internal weather looking like today?
Do I need a hug first, or a sleep or a cry, before I try being kind?
What's my energy level like?

What can I easily do to connect with someone today and speak kindly?
(Perhaps chat to a neighbour, send a random card to a relative,
compliment someone.)

What benefits does kindness give me?
What's my favourite way to be kind?
How can being kind help me in my sobriety?
Because I was sober, this week I . . .

WEEK 8 :
EMOTIONAL TOOLKIT
Understanding the Anger trigger

'I refuse to accept that there's a sort of duality between fact and emotion. If we were to lose the ability to be emotional, if we were to lose the ability to be angry, to be outraged, we would be robots. And I refuse that.'
ARUNDHATI ROY

Summer is associated with the element of fire; we can use it to reignite meaning, purpose and even activism in our lives. This energy brings to mind emotions such as anger, excitement, pride, fear. These are 'high arousal' emotions, meaning that when we are experiencing them the nervous system is activated and the body releases 'action' hormones, such as adrenaline and noradrenaline.

Anger, although often seen negatively, is actually a healthy emotion, signaling to us that something or someone has breached a boundary or hurt us. The tricky part is what to do with it so that we, and others, don't get burnt. As one of the major triggers for drinking and relapse, we need to get tools on board to help us process anger healthily.

There are three ways we can support ourselves and our anger:

1. Learn about healthy boundaries around our time, energy and in our relationships.
2. Recognize and react to what is in our control. A lot of toxic anger comes from fighting battles, the consequences of which we cannot change. If you can, ask yourself, 'What

can I control here?' and let the rest go. We cannot change people, places and things, but we can change how we let them impact us.

3. Find ways to release anger:

- Journal your feelings then destroy/ transform after writing (then you can write whatever you want without fear of recrimination).
- Dance it out – get some rave tunes on or some Nirvana and do your thing.
- Go out to the woods or sit in your car and scream it out.
- Play a racket sport or combat sport.
- Talk to someone (better out than in!).
- Change your surroundings.

NEUROTRANSMITTER HACK: GABA (THE CALMER)

One way to work with anger is to counterbalance it with things that calm and soothe you. Alcohol depletes the natural levels of many neurotransmitters (brain chemicals), in particular GABA (an acronym for gamma-aminobutyric acid), which helps regulate stress and overwhelm. Your brain produces it to facilitate communication between your brain and your nervous system. Known for its calming effects, GABA is your body's main inhibitory neurotransmitter. Its primary job is to inhibit, or reduce, the activity of nerve cells throughout your nervous system. This helps your mind disengage from the alert, wakeful state and transition peacefully into a state of relaxation, and eventually, sleep.[8] You could think of it as a natural anti-anxiety response. It's what we need when the world is spinning to help us calm all the noise.

Alcohol mimics the effects of GABA, which is why so many of us reach for alcohol at the end of the day. It gives us that temporary 'ahhhh . . .' feeling of relaxation. Unfortunately, our brain always searches for homeostasis (balance) and produces less GABA as it thinks alcohol is GABA. (Alcohol is sneaky!) We then have less GABA the day after, and can suffer from a phenomenon known as hangxiety (feeling anxious after drinking), which makes us more likely to reach for alcohol again to soothe this, and thus that terrible cycle starts over.

Maybe you are naturally anxious or a highly sensitive person (we both certainly are) and have used alcohol to soothe anxiety socially – this adds another level of how dependency on alcohol can develop. Alcohol is used to solve a problem and then alcohol becomes the problem.

---

8 Objective Wellness (2021). *How to Increase GABA: 5 Ways to Boost Your Brain's Calming Chemical*. Available at: www.objectivewellness.com/journal/posts/how-to-increase-gaba-5-ways-to-boost-your-brains-calming-chemical

The good news is that there are many ways to develop GABA naturally and help rebalance yourself in the heady, often full-on summer season. Here are some natural ways to help boost your GABA:

Brain food

GABA is produced in your brain from glutamate, an amino acid that is generally abundant in the human diet. It's found in particularly high concentrations in these foods:

- Aged, cured and preserved foods, including cheeses and meats
- Slow-cooked meats and poultry
- Bone broths
- Fish
- Eggs

- Mushrooms
- Tomatoes
- Broccoli
- Walnuts
- Soybeans

In addition to glutamate, your brain requires vitamin B6, to synthesize GABA. So, another way to support GABA production is to increase your intake of vitamin B6 with a multivitamin or B-complex supplement or with B6-rich foods, such as:

- Spinach
- Broccoli
- Brussels sprouts

- Garlic
- Bananas

GABA can also be synthesized in the gut by beneficial bacteria. Eating fermented foods that are rich in probiotics can help to increase GABA levels, for example: [9]

- Sauerkraut
- Kimchi
- Miso

- Tempeh
- Yoghurt
- Kefir

Body Food

Focus on stress-relieving hobbies as they decrease cortisol levels and can increase GABA[10]. Taking just a small amount of exercise on a daily basis, as well as remembering to take walking breaks away

---

9 Food for the Brain (2022). *The Key to a successful Dry January.* Available at: foodforthebrain.org/the-key-to-a-successful-dry-january-the-link-between-alcohol-dependency-and-gaba-deficiency

10 Mikolajczak, M, Gross, JJ & Roskam, I (2019). *Parental Burnout: What Is It, and Why Does It Matter?* Available at: www.researchgate.net/publication/332402868_Parental_Burnout_What_Is_It_and_Why_Does_It_Matter

from the desk or the sofa is enough to help. Slow-paced activities, such as walking outdoors or soft-flow yoga, and activities that regulate the nervous system, such as puzzles, knitting, painting, crafting, swimming and cycling are also good.

Soul food

When we slow down and relax, our nervous system can better regulate and enhance the calming effects of GABA. Try to incorporate some of the following into your regular routine:

- 'Forest bathing' or shinrin-yoku – the mindfulness practice of 'taking in the forest atmosphere' by walking in wooded areas and enjoying your surroundings
- Self-care and rituals (baths, aromatherapy, spa treatments)
- Sensory self-care (listening to calm music, cooking scented foods, moisturizing, looking at pleasing images)
- Listening to a guided meditation (Sarah Blondin and Tara Brach are our faves)

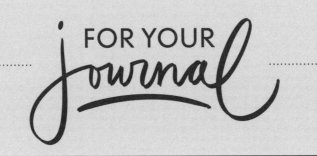

FOR YOUR Journal

What makes you angry? What makes you resentful?
What boundaries are being crossed that make you feel this way?
How can you protect them?
Do you have a way you let your anger out?
What could you do to acknowledge and honour your anger?
What calms you down?
Do you identify as using alcohol to bring down the noise of the day?
What can you do instead?
Because I was sober, this week I . . .

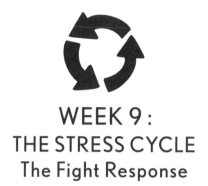

WEEK 9 :
THE STRESS CYCLE
The Fight Response

'It isn't the mountain ahead that wears you out;
it's the grain of sand in your shoe.'
ROBERT W SERVICE

With all the extra activity and longer days we can get really stressed by trying to do it all, be it all and have the most excellent time to make the most of the lovely weather. We cannot address sustainable habit change around problematic drinking without looking at stress and how we respond to it – and the fight response is one of our body's key responses.

Creating strategies in our lives for stress reduction is absolutely key for our wellbeing. Where there is stress and overwhelm there are triggers to drink, so let's lower our stress levels this summer season.

When we tip over into chronic stress and are activated in hyperarousal, it feels like we are under constant threat and so we become incredibly reactive. When we are in states of hyperarousal, such as fight or flight, our body floods with the stress hormone cortisol in order to respond to a threat.

The fight response, when appropriately used, can help you to: find courage and be assertive, establish boundaries, be a leader and protect the ones you love.

However, this response to stress was designed to be activated in a short burst when needed, but many of us find ourselves stuck here, in a constant activated state. This can lead to heightened anxiety, panic, hyperactivity and anger.

This anger often turns inward. We are angry at ourselves for not coping and we give ourselves a really hard time. All these feelings trigger us to search for a coping mechanism and can lead us back to the bottle. This is why building our toolkits and resilience is so important.

TAKING CARE OF OURSELVES IN FIGHT MODE

As with everything we need balance - when stressed or angry we need to release our emotions and self-soothe in self-supportive and helpful ways. We need to return to the idea of nervous system regulation through safety and connection - with exercises to support the Ventral Vagal State (see page 31), where we access the magic of the nervous system to both light us up and calm us down.

Imagine our bodies and minds as a container, which gets filled up with stressors that impact on our nervous system as stress (see image below).

We need healthy coping strategies to act as a tap that we can turn on to release the stress. If we don't do this, the container will get too full and overflow in a meltdown — and however much progress we have made not drinking we end up being triggered to drink as a maladaptive solution to release stress. Alcohol numbs us temporarily, nuking all our neurotransmitters, blocking the tap and becoming the silent yet greatest form of adding to the stress. It depletes our own resilience to cope with the inevitable impactful life experiences we all face.

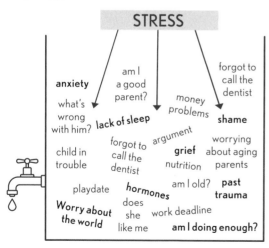

Good coping strategies = tap working – stress release

Not good coping strategies = tap blocked – stress overflows nervous system

NB: vunerability (chronic stress, trauma, build-up of factors) = smaller capacity (window of tolarance) to stress, low resilience

Gathering stress-relieving tools (exercise/breathing, rest, creativity, emotional releases, self-care) enables you to have good coping strategies at your disposal, so you are able to turn on the tap to release the stress when needed.

Keeping hold of bad coping strategies (drinking, ignoring our own needs, people-pleasing, overworking) means the tap gets blocked and stress overflows our nervous system.

Being in stuck in fight mode is a chronic stress state and one ripe for the Wine Witch to come calling and start to wear down your intention to stay sober. We need to check in regularly to look at the big picture and monitor our stress levels.

Stress-relieving checklist:

- ⌀ Identify your particular stressors/triggers (lack of work-life balance, boundaries, environment) and try to make some changes and/or ask for help to address them.
- ⌀ Recognize your vulnerability to that stress at any given time (negative self-talk, perfectionism, impactful life experiences) and be ready rest if your resilience is low.
- ⌀ Remember you can avoid or remove stressors but you must also release the stress from your system, so regular self-care and stress-relieving tools are very important.

Tune in to where you are right now and recognize that at some points your resilience is strong, your energy is high and your ability to cope robust, and yet at other times it's the opposite. We need to work with our natural rhythms rather than battle against them, because otherwise it can lead to burnout and very little residual resilience to avoiding that drink. Summer generally is a season of high energy, which is great, but knowing how to manage it is key.

Self-compassion really is such an important tool: Being stuck in a chronic stress state can leave us feeling ashamed for not coping better. These feelings sink us further into destructive behaviour. One of our all-time favourite mantras from sober forums is 'forgive yourself for what you did when you were still living in survival mode'.

We all have a story of why we ended up relying too heavily on alcohol to a point where we needed to admit it was problematic enough to stop drinking. So, cut yourself some slack, get yourself a sober treat each week to mark your awesome commitment to this fabulous journey, and reach out for help.

Self-compassion also reduces negative self-bias and activates a content and calm state of mind with a disposition for kindness, care, social connectedness and the ability to self-soothe.

Channel your fight response to serve you. We certainly channel it a lot at the alcohol industry these days and their manipulative ways to hoodwink us into thinking a poison is a treat ... Learn your triggers and you'll soon learn to fight for what matters and diffuse it when needed.

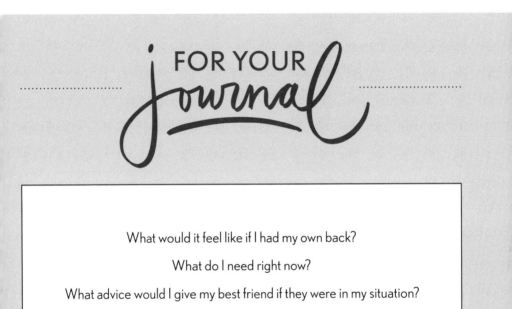

FOR YOUR
Journal

What would it feel like if I had my own back?

What do I need right now?

What advice would I give my best friend if they were in my situation?

What will it take for me to be able to forgive myself?

By holding on to shame who am I serving?

What is one new thing I can do today to treat myself well?

Why do I feel undeserving of feeling well, happy and rested?

How can I be a nurturing adult to myself?

Because I was sober, this week I...

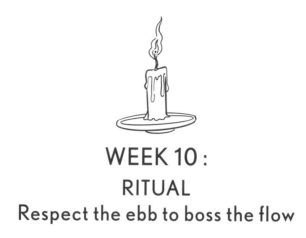

WEEK 10 :
RITUAL
Respect the ebb to boss the flow

'Allow yourself to rest. Your soul speaks to you in the quiet moments in between your thoughts.'
ANON

Summer is the season of busyness. Its energy has a spark of heat to it; with this comes a very real tendency to overexert, take on too much, or load on the pressure to have the 'perfect' summer with the family. When we don't respect our boundaries or needs it can lead to resentment, which can be triggering. If we try to be everything to all people all the time, we end up feeling like nothing is good enough, and this can lead us down a negative spiral of self-talk. As anyone who has spent any time on sober forums will know, 'stinking thinking leads to drinking.' So, this week is all about SERIOUSLY RESTING. We live in a society that doesn't respect or honour rest – it's a huge problem that we delve into in Week 12 – we are stuck in the cult of busy and it's not helping any of us. REST IS BEST – we have learnt to live by the mantra and we hope you will too.

The principle behind the concept of yin and yang is that all things exist as inseparable and contradictory opposites: female-male, dark-light, old-young and so on. The pairs of equal opposites attract and complement each other. Yin energy is the resting, restoring, soothing energy and yang is the fiery, busy, doing energy. We have all become (as has society) totally yangtastic and we need to chill. We need to accept the yin-vitation to take a BLOODY REST. Notice the shouty capitals.

This brings us to our mission statement, 'Respect the ebb to boss the flow', which is our favourite saying of all time and proves that Mandy has a double life as a rapper. If we imagine the flow is the active – the yang – the masculine, the pushing forward, the doing. The ebb is the passive – the yin – the feminine, the receding, the releasing and the being.

If we listen in to our daily, monthly and yearly energy cycles we can avoid being triggered to the fight, flight, freeze or fawn survival states and give ourselves the best chance to get off the autopilot that leads straight down the shop to buy a bottle. WE REPEAT AGAIN, when we are stressed and triggered, any good intentions go out the window as our brain switches to default (glass of wine) to calm down and that is where we get stuck in our drinking thinking, trying to solve a problem with the problem itself.

Training yourself to rest allows your system to reignite itself and kick back into healthy thinking patterns. It helps you move from unconscious survival instincts (old bad habits) back to the new habits you're building around being alcohol-free and your logical and rational mind. It also relates to all the stress, overwhelm and boundary work we have been doing throughout the season, of maintaining and managing ourselves and our energy levels to stay out of the trigger space. Giving time for rest enables us time to replenish and then reignite our creative, inspired and joyful selves.

We cannot give what we don't have, we cannot pour from an empty cup. Become attuned to where you see the ebb and flow. Sit, if you can, and watch the sea. Or turn on Netflix and watch the crackling fire page or seascapes, or put on rain sounds on YouTube. Get still for five minutes and tune in to your breath. Identify times in your day when you can plan a sneaky nap or take an extra three minutes on a coffee break without checking your phone.

Learn how to REST

We all have emergency moments when something triggers us severely and out of the blue. If this happens, try using our acronym, to help yourself through the situation and out the other side.

R - REMOVE yourself from the situation.
E - EXAMINE what's going on for you? What do you really need?
S - SIT and BREATHE deep belly breaths.
T - TRUST that this too shall pass, focus on your breath, and ground yourself in the here and now. Wait until you sigh – that's your sympathetic nervous system coming back online and restoring balance.

Slowing down and taking regular breaks throughout the day is another powerful practice for us to implement because it will help us avoid rising overwhelm levels. If we have become used to using willpower alone to maintain our sobriety, this can weaken over the day as we continue batting away red flags and triggers and holding on by the skin of our teeth. It only takes one straw to break the camel's back and for us to press the F*** It button.

When you respect the ebb – regulate and take time for your energy to restore – you can then boss the flow, those moments which do come in the cycle of summer when you feel full of life and ready to get sh*t done. And you can boss it without burning out in the process.

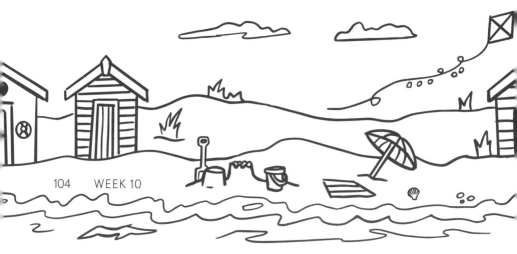

FOR YOUR *journal*

How can I take mini breaks throughout my day?

What could my code word be with my partner/friends when I need a time out?

How restful is my bedroom? What could I do to make it more so?

Where do I feel I can relax?

What can I take off the list this week?

How can I rest more?

Do I have an internal critical voice telling me that being restful is lazy? How can I counteract that voice?

Because I was sober, this week I . . .

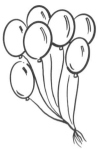

WEEK 11:
THE ART OF SOCIAL
High days and holidays

*'Once a year, go somewhere
you've never been before.'*
THE DALAI LAMA

A key part of what holds people back from changing their relationship with alcohol is the fear that it will be boring and that they will never have fun again, so it's little wonder that summer party time can trigger this fear. The BBQ fires up, the Wine Witch has her flip-flops on, and staying up till 4am at a festival three nights in a row suddenly seems THE BEST IDEA EVER (even though we will feel like death the next day).

Over the last few years there has been a full-on sober and sober-curious revolution. There are great alcohol-free drink alternatives, people are more open to people cutting down or stopping drinking altogether and there are so many sober groups that being sober no longer looks like a social death sentence.

Having said this, high days and holidays (bank holidays/birthdays/cultural celebrations) can still feel heavily drenched in boozy triggers. They have a particular mix of feelings as if it's time out of normal life when normal rules no longer apply. It's all about having a plan and we like an acronym so we made up another one.

If you have any concerns whatsoever about a social occasion and how it might trigger your drinking, make sure you PLAN for it fully in advance:

Prepare Be it a holiday or a party, know what AF drinks there will be, know who will be there, plan what you want to wear and feel like, prepare for the tricky times mentally: the airport, the plane, the first evening (if you get through those things you are winning!). Prepare activities that are not based around booze, like party games or sports activities.

Walk yourself mentally through any event and ask: What am I wearing? What do I smell like? Who am I talking to? What do I drink? What time do I leave? How do I leave? How do I feel when I get home? What do I have planned the next day? How do I reward myself?

Arriving home from a holiday or big social event is often an unexpected trigger, so make sure you have a quiet restorative day planned afterwards with lots of self-care and well-deserved sober treats to manage the social hangover.

Learn Think back to previous events and what you have learned from them. What is like for you in these heightened situations? How easy has it been to manage your drinking before? What are your triggers? How can you protect yourself? Take quit lit and podcasts with you on holiday to keep you engaged in your alcohol-free choice.

Aspire Keep future-focused: play it forward, and think about how proud you will be as you become a morning bird who savours the empty beach or gets up and goes to yoga when everyone else is in bed with a hangover.

Notice Stay curious about your environment, yourself and your experience. What's different about it when you're not drinking? Are there new places to discover? People to talk to? Foods to eat? What do you notice about your mood and your needs?

Many of us put off stopping drinking because of a forthcoming event. We think, 'I can't possibly quit before Christmas', or, 'I have my best friend's wedding coming up', but there will always be more occasions or events so ask yourself, why does drinking play such a central role? There is never a socially convenient, 'good' time to stop, but there is never a bad time to stop either. We have never met anyone who has regretted quitting the booze, but we have certainly met many who have regretted continuing.

It can be really useful, especially in the early days, to flip your thinking around what it means to be social when you are on holiday. To focus on mornings – breakfasts and brunches, sunrises and sports, walks and papers and lying in the sun without a hangover. Some people might see being sober as a state of deprivation because we don't do that one thing. But, in fact, it is the exact opposite – because we don't do that one thing we get to do EVERYTHING else. Rather than waiting all day for the drinking to start, or getting over the pain of the night before, we get to have the whole day ahead of us. We get to benefit from, and be present in, every moment. At a wedding you get to feel the love, at a party you get to actually connect with people, on holiday you ACTUALLY RELAX!

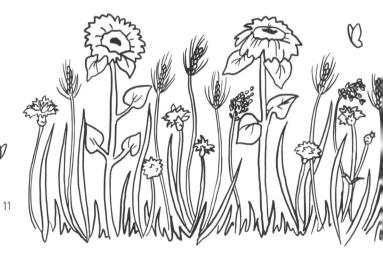

FOR YOUR *Journal*

What worries me about high days and holidays being alcohol-free?

What do I need to PLAN?

When I play it forward and see myself drinking, and see myself the day after, what is the picture?

How does it differ if I'm not drinking?

Where would I like to discover that I have never been?

Because I was sober, this week I . . .

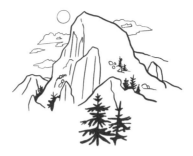

WEEK 12 :
THE SCHOOL OF LIFE
The Cult of Busy

'Beware the barrenness of a busy life.'
SOCRATES

It seems we are on the go 24/7, we cross the road faster than we used to, we rarely unplug, many of us find it increasingly difficult to switch off and we feel guilty if we do so. We are living within the Cult of Busy. The summer energy feeds this with extra socializing, longer days, summer holidays and the periods of school closure. We have expectations of fun in the sun and making the most out of every day and, often, every night too.

The Cult of Busy is no joke. Parental burnout – 'an exhaustion syndrome, characterized by feeling physically and mentally overwhelmed' by being a parent has been studied by Belgian psychologists Isabelle Roskam and Moïra Mikolajczak[11]. With the increase of working from home and home schooling during the pandemic, it made its way into the headlines of national newspapers and glossy mags alike. The glorification of multi-tasking – which women are so good at (eye roll) – is a mental health issue. It also affects memory and productivity. The Cult of Busy (COB) leaves us with stress activation in the sympathetic nervous system (fight/flight) which means, for example, we can't digest food and repair ourselves effectively so our bodies, minds and spirits struggle and eventually break down. We can feel overwhelmed, exhausted, hopeless and detached.

---

11 https://www.researchgate.net/publication/332402868_Parental_Burnout_What_Is_It_and_Why_Does_It_Matter

The COB also plays havoc with our hormonal health, as it does not respect the cyclical energy fluctuations we have around our menstrual cycles or the transitions to motherhood or into the menopause. These can impact on our mental and emotional health – which in turn impacts our habit to imbibe alcohol as a 'stress reliever' and is why women report spikes in drinking around these rites of passage.

Planning here is key – blocking out time, not only for exercise and hobbies but also the boring stuff like the tax return and the washing AND time to do sweet FA.

We have got into the habit of seeing activities as valid only if they are productive. We have to start allocating time for proper, intentional rest and restore time. We also need time to reflect, to sit and stare into space. We cannot be on the go all the time.

If you find yourself starting to rush, use that as a little flag to point you back to taking a pause, a few breaths, a break to pace and calm yourself. Outsource anything you can afford to outsource. Identify the hugest pain in your butt and outsource that – you could use the money you save on alcohol to get support. Ask for help from loved ones so you can take time to have a bubble bath or a blissful walk ALONE. Having help is something neither of us considered – we had to do it all and be it all. For generations women's worth was tied up with how well we kept all those plates spinning. Not anymore, no way José. The gaff is up and we call BS.

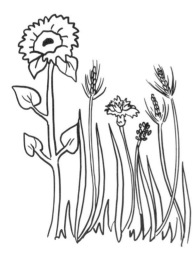

I had a good look at the domestic overwhelm and identified that the washing load was the straw that broke this camel's back, so I found a lady locally who now does my ironing and it is a life-changer. It is returned to me in neat piles and makes me feel like someone is taking care of me. I am super grateful to her and we have now become friends. KATE

I had a very strong narrative that self-care was being selfish, asking for help was a failure and resting was lazy. I got entangled in some concept of feminism that if I didn't do it all really well all by myself then the patriarchy would win and pack me back off to the kitchen. In reality, no one can do life alone. We all need support – companies have whole structures of hierarchal support, players in a football team support each other – we succeed when we work together. I had a real sense of martyrdom – that to be a good parent I had to self-sacrifice and do everything for everyone at the expense of my own wellbeing, but nobody was asking me to do that. Being able to say, 'Help! I am struggling here, I need support,' isn't a weakness, it's a strength. MANDY

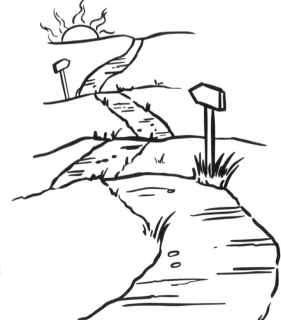

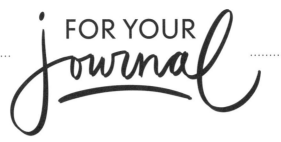

FOR YOUR Journal

Am I stuck in the Cult of Busy?

How can I cultivate a narrative of self-care NOT
as selfish but as essential?

What advice would I give my best friend if they were doing all the things I do?

How can I be my own best friend here?

What can I delegate?

What can I outsource?

Because I was sober, this week I . . .

WEEK 13 :
TOOLS FOR GREATER REFLECTION
Your emergency toolkit

'Confidence comes from being prepared.'
JOHN WOODEN

Like all good girl scouts we need to be prepared for when the sh*t hits the fan, which it invariably will, especially over the summer and, for the mums, in the period of school closure, which they in all their darkness and sinister humour call 'the school holidays.' Mwahahahaha. The house will be a disaster, it will all get too much, we will scream and cry and eat ice cream, but WE WILL NOT DRINK. We do need a plan though. This is our guide to an emergency toolkit, those practices you can reach to when needed to cool those (school holiday?) beans.

Using our favourite HALT acronym, check in with yourself and take a break when things get too much:

Hungry – Eat something. Drink water!
Angry – Punch a cushion, go for a run.
Lonely – Phone a friend who respects and supports your sober journey, log on to a sober group – they will always understand and talk you through a trigger time.
Tired – Lie down, get some rest, have an early night, put on a film for your kids. Get outside, bathe in dappled light under a tree.

It can be all too easy to get caught up in summer comparison-itis, which can get us down and make us feel like we aren't enough. Remember you ARE enough, and you are worth staying in your own lane and bossing your own game as a supersoberstar.

Perhaps you're dealing with guilt as your kids are at the crèche, which they hate, because you have to work, or everyone seems to be having a GREAT time and your kids are having a TV-tastic holiday as money is tight and every activity, theme park and attraction is SO expensive. All of this can impact your self-esteem, wear you down and be a trigger.

Emergency toolkit self-esteem boosters:

- Don't get caught up in the beach body diet BS, because all bodies are beach bodies.
- Take a social media break to cut out the noise of others.
- Speak kindly to yourself, wear clothes that make you feel special.
- Go to the party or don't go to the party – remember you are in control.

For your self-care, some honesty and some support is needed. Perhaps hold a family meeting, talk to family members about how you are feeling, delegate housekeeping tasks, make a plan for a special day with each child. Be mindful of age-appropriate activities. We have certainly wasted money on taking kids to places when they were too young and lacked the capacity to really experience them. Be mindful of over-committing and aware of family triggers. Remember your boundaries and use them.

As much as it is a time to protect ourselves from triggers, and rest, this summer season is also the time to look outward and reignite our joy in the little things we missed by being hungover, depleted or depressed when we chose alcohol over ourselves. It's exciting to think about the new hope and possibility we can harness using the summer energy to move into action. What can you start anew? A morning ritual, perhaps, or long walks in the late summer sunshine without thinking about drinking, just being present and really feeling the joys of your new sober lease of life.

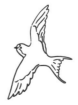

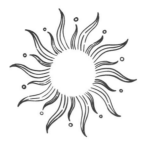

SUMMER SOLSTICE
Ritual and reflection

'Bask in this blessed light, lie amidst daisies and sand. Sun Enlivening.'
CHARLOTTE BRONTË

The summer solstice is a powerful planetary moment when the tilt of the Earth brings us closest to the sun. The longest day of the year provides an absolute abundance of rich fire energy we can use to inspire, uplift and energize us.

This is a zenith – a moment of glory, and a great time to focus in on the power that sobriety gives us, the force of intention, the bloody-mindedness of going against the grain. We burned away the dross of others' expectations and opinions and can now bask in the sunshine of the wellbeing we are creating for ourselves. We feel like winners. We are winners, we have gone for gold!

This super social season was, for many of us, a peak time of drinking socially, and a lot of effort has gone into reframing this period and creating new habits. We may have had some sadness or nostalgia around the occasions we associate with alcohol, so we can use the metaphor of the sun, shining a clear light on those associations, to remember hangovers in the heat and to use the clarity and purpose that comes with this energy to stoke the sober flame in us to keep strong.

It's also important to pause, reflect and really own this achievement of sustaining our efforts and sobriety. After the solstice, the Earth continues on its cycle and begins tilting away from the sun, and the days start growing shorter again. We're already beginning the shift inward. The days will continue to shorten until the Winter Solstice and we begin the cycle of growth all over again. This season our zest for life has been reignited in sobriety and we can capture these feelings and conserve them for the when we move into the more reflective seasons of autumn and winter.

SUMMER SOLSTICE SUN RITUALS

We invite you to perform a ritual to honour the passage of time at the solstice, and to use it as a time to pause and reflect. You can light a fire, watch the sunset, sunbathe, light candles – whatever way you tune in to the energy of the heat and the sun, take a moment to really enjoy it. At this time of ritual, note your inner highlight reel: what are your proudest moments of bossing it sober, coping with a challenge or setting boundaries this season?

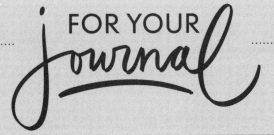

FOR YOUR *Journal*

What were my wins?
What challenges did I overcome?
What am I proud of?
How will I reward myself?
What is my sober power mantra?
What passion have I reignited that I will take forward
with me in autumn?
If I secretly knew the answer – what would it be?
Because I was sober, this week I . . .

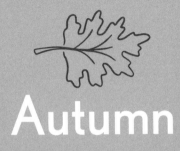

Autumn

'Every leaf speaks bliss to me
Fluttering from the autumn tree.'
EMILY BRONTË

HARNESSING THE POWER OF THE GIFTS OF AUTUMN TO REWRITE

Autumn is a beautiful season. It is a time of mists and the end of harvests, with treasures like conkers and berries tempting us outside to get that vitamin D before the winter sets in. Autumn is like a fabulous old drag queen, doing her last public performance, determined to go out with a bang. Let's celebrate that queen!

And as we enter autumn and the days shorten, we start the REWRITE phase of our R4 Balance Method. As the animals prepare for colder, darker months, so do we. It's a time to simplify, release and nurture in preparation for the essentials we need for winter. This is nature's edit, when we look at letting go of what no longer serves us, like the trees shedding leaves making room for fresh growth. We let go of alcohol and make room for the gift of sober living; this refining process continues like the endless tide polishing a pebble.

There is a natural turning inward we feel in the autumn, a greater inclination toward introversion as we retreat indoors, start to light fires (or put on the central heating), and get on the knitwear. This is an ideal time to nurture creativity, try new hobbies, get the slow cooker out, watch box sets or get into an old classic novel. Whether we have kids, or still indulge our inner kid, we may love this season's high days of Halloween and, in the UK, Bonfire Night.

Autumn needs its own special recipe for self-care, to replenish us. At this time of year, we are often running on empty after the summer, while simultaneously handling back-to-school admin and emotions. If we have kids, they are back to school and so often we may be trying to play catch-up at work, without even drawing breath. After the busyness and sociability of the summer we may feel like we need a holiday! Sometimes drinking triggers can be strong as we have held on with willpower through the high energy of summer – the crash afterwards leads to depletion and wanting to drink.

How does this season affect you? Are you all about jumping in leaves, excited about boots and knitwear? Do you yearn to get out to a deer park and read Jane Eyre for the 50th time? Or are you more reflective at this time of year? Do you tend to feel a lowering of mood as the nights draw in? As Hippocrates said, 'Look to the season when choosing your cures.' It's about knowing how you tick and what you need.

Return to this section when you feel the need to practise acceptance, release things that no longer serve you or rewrite what you need with the darkening days.

REASONS TO BE CHEERFUL IN AUTUMN

Jumpers and woolly scarves, new perfume, hot chocolate, cinema dates, coffee and cake, hot yoga, stews, collecting conkers and mini pumpkins, film nights, cuddles, muddy walks, new sheepskin slippers, candles, fairy lights

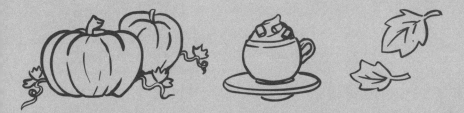

──── FOR YOUR JOURNAL ────

How do I want to feel this autumn?

What matters to me the most this season?

When do I feel happiest/calm/joyful?

What would I like to create or nurture in my life this season?

Which elements make autumn special for me?

What fears would I like to release this autumn?

Because I was sober, this week I . . .

WEEK 1:
YOUR SEASONAL PLANNER

'A goal without a plan is just a wish.'
ANTOINE DE SAINT-EXUPÉRY

Let's have a look at the overview of your autumn. As with every season, we are designing our life map according to the natural features and lay of the land and planning our route to better prepare for our journey. What holidays or extra family commitments do you have coming up? What challenges might they bring? Is it a heavy work season? How can you take things off the list? What fun things have you got to look forward to? Too many?

Fill in your simple planner to note your intentions for specific dates and some questions for deeper reflection to get your autumn hygge on!

AUTUMN
Planner

Month 1

Month 2

Month 3

Hobbies to try ....

....

....

Key dates

Possible Triggers

Strategy ....
Movement ....
Self-care ....

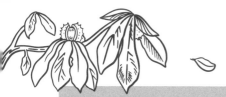

HOW TO USE YOUR PLANNER FOR AUTUMN

Look through your diary and pick out the days that are family birthdays, major festivals or national bank holidays. Plan for when you will need to self-protect your sober choice the most.

If this is your first sober autumn, how can you snuggle in to this delicious season?

Adjust your self-care to suit the autumn energy. Do you feel like changing up your exercise? Maybe getting some spice into your diet or changing your wardrobe to suit the shift in seasons?

Check in with your feelings about this time of year. As with the other seasons, we challenge you to:

- Try a new alcohol-free drink
- Read a new book
- Do a new hobby or activity that you have always wanted to try
- Say no to something you don't want to do
- Add in some movement
- Add in some self-care

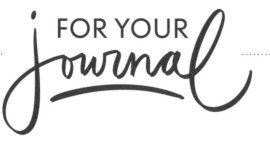

FOR YOUR Journal

What associations do I have with these major dates coming up?

How confident on a scale of 1–10 do I feel about managing this period alcohol-free?

Which activities do I want to opt out of this year?

What key dates have I identified that are important to me?

How do they normally relate to drinking alcohol?

What new rituals can I introduce?

Are there certain dates I need to plan around because of alcohol?

What will I do?

What do I need to do to increase my confidence level by 1 point?

(Have a friend there, opt out, drive, journal more, get a coach?)

What might I do instead?

What might I drink instead?

What can I plan in instead?

Because I was sober, this week I . . .

What is your confidence level now from 1-10? Hopefully it will have improved.

If not, go back and see if you can generate more options.

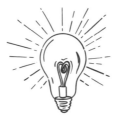

WEEK 2 :
SETTING YOUR INTENTION
Letting go

'When I let go of what I am, I become what I might be.'
FROM TAO TE CHING

Autumn provides us with the perfect example of the art of letting go. We grow through our life cycles and release old versions of ourselves, outdated habits and old perceptions of ourselves that have held us back and kept us stuck. Just as the trees shed their leaves to nourish the earth and allow for new growth, so do our own patterns of acceptance and release.

Sometimes this process is so gradual we don't realize we are changing. As adults we often feel static and don't notice the shedding of skin, the liminal periods and our gradual growth over time. Sometimes, however, we can be forced to let go of something by a life event or rite of passage, such as a bereavement or becoming a mother, and we must adapt to survive, sink or swim.

So, we know that it isn't always easy to accept and release. Reclaiming power and control has significance for many of us as women – and if we have experienced trauma or abuse the need for control is even more charged. It can be frightening to loosen our grip because being in control may have made us feel safe. We may not even know how to let go. There is a lot of energy spent holding onto the past and to things that aren't working, so we find ourselves on the edge of the precipice - we can't go back and yet we are too scared to take a leap of faith.

There is relief in accepting the things we can't change, and the struggle is often in the process of reaching that point. When we realize that we are done with alcohol and that it was never going to be good for us, that fight is over. With this acceptance comes a tsunami of other acceptances and the letting go of many things that we didn't anticipate. We find we can also let go of the expectations of our own perfection that led us to dial down our stress with booze, and we can let go of shoehorning ourselves into events and friendships that aren't good for us. We let go of a version of ourselves and make way for who we are now. We literally get to rewrite a new story of our future.

By letting go of something that no longer serves us, we become stronger and more empowered. Through letting go, we actually gain control.

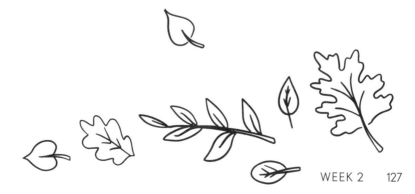

HOW TO LET GO WITH SELF-COMPASSION

When we let go, and call attention to things that don't serve us anymore, we bring mindful scrutiny to the sore spots and for this it's essential we learn to use self-compassion. Think of something you wish to let go of – it might be perfectionism, rushing, or a habit such as going to bed too late – and then apply the following:

- First, create a positive mantra to counteract any painful thoughts that may arise, and keep a journal to help you process change gradually.
- Create physical distance or a safe space to process any feelings that occur, and avoid situations that trigger you around this subject until you are stronger.
- Practise mindfulness and self-compassion to keep bringing yourself back to the present moment with love rather than getting stuck in a cycle of rumination.
- Be gentle with yourself.
- Know that it's OK not to be OK and find ways to release negative emotions rather than ignoring them or keeping them bottled up. Remember your tools such as movement, journaling or connecting with others.
- Remember you can't control others – only your own response.
- Seek out people who understand you and inspire you, make you feel positive and help you see the lighter side of life.
- Give yourself permission to talk about what's bothering you with friends, family or support groups, or to seek professional help.
- Look for your joy. Keep being curious about what you love and what excites and nourishes you.

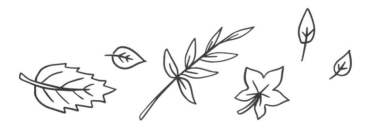

FOR YOUR *Journal*

What or who is
no longer
serving me?

What would
I like to do
instead?

What do I
like now?

How can I love
myself a bit
more today?

How will I
know when it
is working?

Which affirmations or mantras can I use?
For example: *I am trying my best, I deserve to be loved. I was doing the best I could.*
Because I was sober, this week I . . .

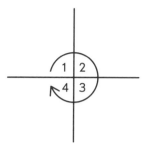

WEEK 3:
CYCLES AND SOBRIETY
The Stages of Change explained

'I can't change the direction of the wind,
but I can adjust my sails to always reach my destination.'
JIMMY DEAN

The Stages of Change model from the works of Prochaska and DiClemente is one of the fundamental models professionals use in understanding the process of changing habits and behaviour. It has much in common with the Panarchic theory (see page 2), and its stages can be seen as seasons, with their different energies and challenges.

Once we have left what's called the 'precontemplative stage' where we are only subconsciously aware of the need to change, our journey begins. After our first contemplation or sober curiosity that begun in our sober winter, come the preparations of spring. Then the action of change in summer moves into the deeper autumnal cycle of maintenance, with practices to sustain these changes before we cycle back to rest and reflect in winter. Then, the pattern starts once again as we move into the next year, the next cycle of change in our lives and our alcohol-free journey, each year getting easier, and ourselves becoming braver and more expansive as time goes on.

THE STAGES OF CHANGE CYCLE

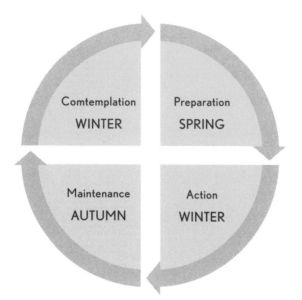

This non-linear approach reflected our own personal sober journeys and those of many of the women we work with. Many of us had cycled around and entered the contemplative stage of going sober more than once, and more than once returned to drinking. Perhaps it started with a 3am Google search, 'Am I an alcoholic?' or a visit to the doctors that felt uncomfortable when we had to fill in the number of units we drank. Then, we may have gone back to drinking. We had prepared – we read a book, listened to a podcast, but then went back to the vino habit. We had taken action – both of us had long periods of sobriety – but the allure of the old associations of alcohol, or stress had called us back to drinking. It took us many, many years to get to the maintenance stage, which is why we would never risk, take for granted or forget how far we have come, and it's why we keep working at the maintenance on our sober fields.

We are not advocating that people go back to drinking after a period of sobriety in the name of learning. For us, those periods were the hardest of our sober journeys. We often felt like we were playing Russian roulette with our health and our safety. It only takes one fatal blackout for drinking to take an incredibly dangerous turn and we often sighed in relief waking up from that night when we had gone too far, knowing that we were lucky nothing worse had happened.

Of course, some of us have only one Day 1 – something sticks, the decision is made and hard work and favourable conditions make it work. We wish this for everyone and if we could have managed it ourselves it would have spared us heartache, wasted opportunities and fear, but it is what it is and there is no shame in the struggle. It is, as they say, a journey and not a destination.

If you are returning to alcohol-free living, it is your choice to frame this in the way that is most empowering to you. Although we both have a 'Continuous Sober Date' starting with the last Day 1, sometimes we both talk about our sober journeys in longer terms – from the first time we both engaged with the process of enquiry and recovery, despite returning to drinking after a year sober – because we want to honour the learning inherent in getting up, falling down and trying again.

Whatever this journey looks like for you, to have got from where you were to where you are now takes tenacity and courage, and we salute you. We found it helpful to understand that this cyclical process is often part of the story of a 'grey-area drinker', and that for many of us it's a case of three steps forward and one step back in order to take that final leap. Hopefully, this model of change provides some greater understanding about our behaviours and helps us realize that our attempts are not failure but learning. So, keep on keeping on – you are amazing!

Now, for us, the Stages of Change model encompasses wider aspects of our lives, not just not drinking. As the years pass free from alcohol, so does the scope of our recovery and growth, and being able to live our lives fully and learn is a true gift.

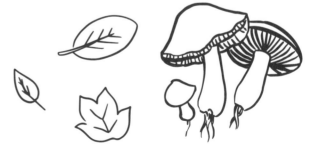

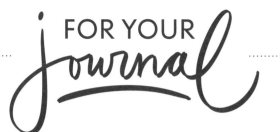

FOR YOUR journal

How can I harness the Stages of Change model to help me?

Which part do I find the most difficult?

What else in my life would I like to change?

What does preparation look like for me?

How can I take action?

What do I need to be able to maintain the changes I would like to make?

Because I was sober, this week I . . .

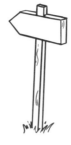

WEEK 4:
CULTIVATING SOBER SPACE
Affirmations

'There is nothing either good or bad,
but thinking makes it so.'
WILLIAM SHAKESPEARE

Affirmations are short phrases we can use to boost our mood. No longer just the territory of yoga lovers and self-help fans, they are now commonplace throughout business, sport and coaching as a performance strategy. Positive affirmations begin with 'I am . . .'. We state something in the present as if it is already true. By repeating these regularly, we begin to bring them into our conscious thought and, as with anything else, repetition over time becomes a habit and part of our unconscious mind.

Autumn is a great time to focus on cultivating an affirmation practice. As we begin to enter the darker times of the year we want to nourish ourselves with warming foods and seek out comfort, so our thoughts need to reflect this. Affirmations are like the blankets and hot water bottles of our thought processes, keeping us warm and insulated from the harsh outside conditions of 24-hour news cycles, cultural expectations and the negative biases of our own minds.

Neuroscientists endorse affirmations as proven methods of self-improvement because of their ability to rewire our brains. Affirmations, much like exercise, raise the level of feel-good hormones and push our brains to form new clusters of positive thought neurons[12]. In the sequence of thought-speech-action, affirmations play an integral role by breaking patterns of negative thought, negative speech and, in turn, negative actions.

We like to see them as little spells whispered at the Wine Witch to give protection against her BS, and as an antidote to the undermining influence of the inner critic who often sabotages our attempts to embrace our power and keep going with our goals. You may identify with us in that keeping yourself small, or playing down your strengths, was an adaptive survival strategy that kept you safe/accepted/liked in your life. One thing's for sure – we all have the inner voice that we wish would shut up – and many of us drank to make it go quiet.

For many of us, the insidious negative self-talk shows up in unhealthy perfectionism, low expectations and a mindset of being never-quite-good-enough. As women, we miss opportunities because, say, we expect ourselves to be perfect before we accept that speaking gig. We don't challenge someone in a boardroom who nicks our ideas. Perhaps we put others first all the time, because we think that love is the same as self-sacrifice. Or we bash ourselves constantly for every mistake we have made, which keeps us stuck in a vicious cycle of self-harming thoughts and behaviours. Affirmations and positive self-talk can be a powerful tool in our arsenal to counteract our negative bias and society's gender bias.

Every minute of every day, our bodies are physically changing in response to the thoughts that run through our heads. When we practise gratitude, we get a surge of rewarding neurotransmitters, like dopamine and norepinephrine, and experience a general uplift in mood. So, positive thinking is like a muscle, a habit that gets stronger with practise, and affirmations are bite-size anchors to moor the mind efficiently. Just thinking about something causes your brain to send signals and release neurotransmitters. These chemicals control virtually all of your body's functions, including your mood and feelings. Over time and with repetition, it's been proven that your thoughts change your brain, your cells, and even your genes. They are indeed magic. You can work creatively with this repetition too – put affirmations on Post-it notes around the house, change your passwords on your computer, make Pinterest boards, download the *I am* app, repeat them out loud.

---

12 Taylor, AR PhD (2022). *Affirmations.* Available at:www.arlenetaylor.org/brain-care/953-affirmation

SOBER AFFIRMATIONS:

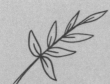

I am sober.
I am sober and the rest is good enough.
I am a sober badass.
I am living a life I choose without alcohol.
I am free of alcohol.
I am choosing to make my mental and physical health a priority.

DEFEATING THE INNER CRITIC AFFIRMATIONS:

I am proud of myself.
I am trying my best.
I am worthy of my dreams.
I am able to change.
I am ready for a new day.
I am capable.
I am stronger than I think.
I am a good mum.

KATE'S FAVES:

I am sober and the rest is good enough.
I haven't come this far to only come this far.

MANDY'S FAVES:

I am worthy of love and to be loved.
I am my own best friend.
It is what it is, so move on.

FOR YOUR *journal*

How did I feel reading about affirmations?

Was there resistance to this idea? Why might this be?

What sober affirmation will I use?

In what areas of my life do I hear that critical voice the most?

What positive affirmations can I find to help me in this specific area?

Because I was sober, this week I . . .

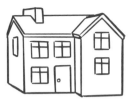

WEEK 5:
BOSSING YOUR ENVIRONMENT
Hygge

'Sanity is a cosy life.'
SUSAN SONTAG

Hygge, or the Danish art of happiness, hit the mainstream in 2018. Spoken aloud, this little word that sounds a bit like a hug – 'hue-ga' – means 'a quality of cosiness and comfortable conviviality that engenders a feeling of contentment or wellbeing,' and is regarded as a defining characteristic of Danish culture. According to Hyggehouse.com, another definition of hygge is, 'an art of creating intimacy', either with yourself, friends or your home. While there's no one English word or simple definition to describe hygge, several can be used interchangeably, including cosiness, charm, happiness, contentedness, security, familiarity, comfort, reassurance, kinship and simplicity.

If hygge was a photo, it would be woolly socks, or a hot chocolate with a friend or loved one in front of a roaring fire. As the nights are starting to draw in, we need those treats, rewards and care to keep the spirits up so we don't try to find comfort in booze. This Nordic way of embracing the darker months has so much to teach us in the way of respecting the ebb of our lives as opposed to always expecting to be on the go or in 'flow', and about finding the joy in those darker times by nurturing ourselves with seasonal intent.

Getting some seasonal treats on board helps us ward off the temptation of the fantasy of mulled wine in front of the fire. We need to intentionally adopt new rituals and routines, and hygge is a great roadmap for autumn and winter habit hacks.

It's been said that you can't buy hygge. Many have waxed lyrical about its essence and grumbled about it becoming a lifestyle trend. However, according to Meik Weiking, Director at The Institute of Happiness in Copenhagen, you don't need to be too worthy about it. Weiking suggests that some simple ways to begin to adopt hygge can be bought: 'Light candles and eat more cakes,' he says. We are SO down with that. He also says we need to wear tracky bottoms more often and stay in. Reader, we may marry him, in fact. If that all feels a bit Covid lockdown right now, just remember it's a choice – it's about balancing out periods of high socializing, busy work periods and over-exertion with downtime, cosiness and calm.

The Danes created hygge as a way to survive and thrive during the autumn and winter months and acknowledged that by simplifying and becoming present we can dramatically affect our emotional and mental wellbeing. By using simple practices, they found ways of bringing warmth and connection in a highly intentional way to lift the spirits. Hygge is not a big feasting high moment, a 'go hard or go home' party binge; it's a daily sprinkling of warmth and care over our environment, our communities, our homes and the people we love, a symbol of gathering round a fire to huddle and be together. Simple rituals to attend with care to the everyday, like lighting a candle with each meal, or mindfully drinking your cinnamon latte in front of a fire, is embracing the spirit of hygge.

This Danish art of cultivating happiness and wellbeing calls attention to the small things that we too can bring our attention to in our environment. Hygge asks us to engage with, turn toward, accept and find joy in this activity. It also encourages a mindful approach to when we want to connect and also retreat. For those of us who are more introverted, hygge says 'brunch with your bestie is good enough.' We are allowed to go small, opt out and nurture ourselves in ways that feel cosy and cheerful.

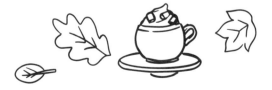

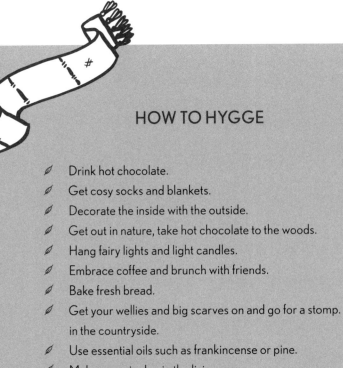

HOW TO HYGGE

- Drink hot chocolate.
- Get cosy socks and blankets.
- Decorate the inside with the outside.
- Get out in nature, take hot chocolate to the woods.
- Hang fairy lights and light candles.
- Embrace coffee and brunch with friends.
- Bake fresh bread.
- Get your wellies and big scarves on and go for a stomp. in the countryside.
- Use essential oils such as frankincense or pine.
- Make a movie den in the living room.
- Eat soups and stews.

FOR YOUR *journal*

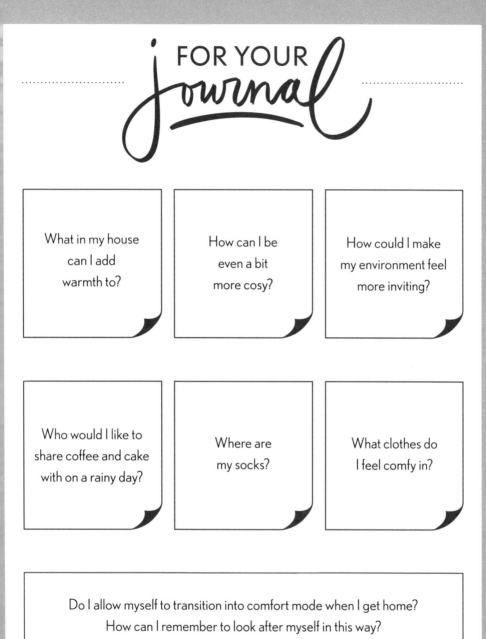

What in my house
can I add
warmth to?

How can I be
even a bit
more cosy?

How could I make
my environment feel
more inviting?

Who would I like to
share coffee and cake
with on a rainy day?

Where are
my socks?

What clothes do
I feel comfy in?

Do I allow myself to transition into comfort mode when I get home?
How can I remember to look after myself in this way?
Because I was sober, this week I . . .

WEEK 6 :
RESEARCHING OUR RESOURCES
Rewriting creativity and hobbies

'Delicious autumn! My very soul is wedded to it,
and if I were a bird I would fly about the Earth
seeking the successive autumns.'
GEORGE ELIOT

Autumn is a season that has inspired creatives across the globe for centuries' possibly because of its beautiful colours and the tension between the fullness of harvest and the melancholy that can come with the ebb and the letting go as we enter the darker months. Vincent Van Gogh, Georgia O'Keeffe, Claude Monet and Higashiyama Kaii are just a few who have been inspired to capture its hues and tones in visual art. Emily Brontë famously loved autumn, writing how 'every leaf speaks bliss to me, fluttering from the autumn tree,' and this sumptuous season is of course immortalized by Keats as, 'The season of mists and mellow fruitfulness.'

Autumn also lends itself to creative endeavour from us less lofty folks and encourages us into gentler pastimes and hobbies as we naturally retreat inside and seek out activities to occupy ourselves. In the SMART Recovery (Self-Management And Recovery Training) model, which is an alternative to the 12-step fellowship model, members are encouraged to have a VACI (a Vital Absorbing Creative Interest), such is the importance of creativity in creating a place of flow and peace when disengaging from addictive substances and behaviours. When we engage creatively and are absorbed, the mind is stilled and the internal chatter that is so hard to manage in the early days goes quiet for a while. Flow is that sweet spot between creative thinking or problem solving and losing yourself in an activity.

Creativity takes countless forms: it could be in writing your journal or reading this book! It could be photography, knitting, painting, crafting, playing computer games or doing Sudoku, it could be gardening or flower arranging or organizing your house. You may not see playing tennis as being creative, but you are in fact accessing your creative brain to set up shots, analyse the game of your opponent and move your body accordingly. There are literally thousands of different hobbies out there to explore. By engaging in different activities we rewrite the shape of our day, consciously creating new ways of being. Check out our website for some ideas: www.lovesober.com.

Each new season is an opportunity to look at the everyday afresh. What is the sense of the season? What is its mood, its colours, its timbre? What are its smells, its rituals, its high days? Autumn is a season of curating and rewriting, discerning the priorities we want to take forward and the fat that can be trimmed. You could go through your phone and delete the thousands of pictures you don't want and print the best ones for a scrapbook or photo album. You might find yourself reading more, writing journals, getting the urge to use lights and colours, and changing your food to colourful roots and hotpots. Collecting vibrant leaves and conkers may appeal to your inner child.

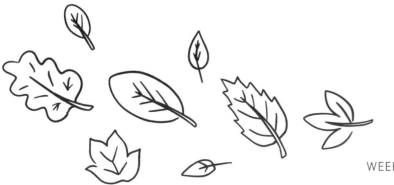

How can you mindfully approach your day and engage with nature creatively?

Perhaps you could experiment with painting or wood- or pumpkin-carving this autumn, or begin to play with fashion and colour in a creative way. Do you notice the shadows lengthening? How does the chill in the morning and woodsmoke remind you of old times or stories? Try journaling this. Download a filming app on your phone, capture an autumn walk and put some music to it.

We do not have to be a Brontë or an O'Keeffe to create. Part of being creative is the element of play, the unknown and getting messy. We are allowed to be really rubbish at things and do them just for the hell of it. We can be grand, messy amateurs and embrace the true spirit and freedom of being amateurs – after all, the word 'amateur' itself comes from the French 'for the love of'. Imagine the unbridled joy of making mud pies, dancing like no one can see us, and yelling Abba tunes at the top of our lungs with noise reducing headphones on so we can't even hear ourselves . . . Now we're talking.

FOR YOUR *journal*

How do I love to
be creative?

What do I never do
that I could try?

What did I used to do
that I no longer do?

What would I
never do?

What's my favourite
autumn book?

What would I love
to do on a rainy day?

Who could I write a
letter to and how
might I make it really
colourful?

What would I do if
I wasn't bothered
about the mess?

What happens if I let
go of it being 'good'?

Because I was sober, this week I . . .

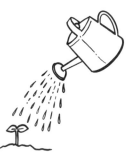

WEEK 7 :
FOSTERING POSITIVE GROWTH
Gratitude

"'Enough" is a feast.'
BUDDHIST PROVERB

Gratitude – the feeling of thankful appreciation for favours or benefits received – is a fundamental tenet of traditional pathways of sobriety, expounded in 12-step philosophy and studied for eons in the fields of ethics and philosophy. It has become a common topic in lifestyle magazines and self-help books alike. Because of its mighty reputation, we had to look closely at this virtue to understand its seemingly magical properties.

Gratitude is about the ability to notice and tune in to everyday things in our lives. These are things we often overlook but, with practise, noticing them, turning toward them and naming them help fill up our cup throughout the day and boost our mood significantly. So, first we have to stop and pause, then we get curious and then we ask our minds to focus in on something that we feel thankful for and sit with it for a while, dwelling on it and feeling it in our bodies.

In truth, the practice of gratitude can be like an inoculation against negativity.

Focusing on the gifts we have in our lives counteracts our negative bias and reminds us that even when bad things happen there is still good in the world and in our lives. It cultivates the 'glass half full' mentality and halts the 'stinking thinking that leads to drinking.'

To make gratitude work it needs to be done regularly, like building a muscle, but it also needs to be done with novelty. This means thinking of new things we are grateful for each day rather than bringing to mind the same things over and over. This is because our brains quickly adapt to anything that stays constant. They go looking for the next special thing. By mixing it up and focusing on things we are grateful for, we're constantly giving our brains something new and positive to focus on.

Studies into the benefits of gratitude show that it boosts self-esteem and connections because it reduces social comparison. Rather than becoming resentful toward people who have more money or better jobs, grateful people are able to appreciate other people's accomplishments while feeling they are and have enough. These relational parts of the brain are so important in maintaining sobriety and wellbeing.

We suggest at least once a week you write a gratitude list for being alcohol-free. It never gets old to wake up each day hangover-free and it's worth acknowledging it. To super-boost your gratitude practice you can share out loud with others why you are grateful and appreciate them; this helps us to strengthen those connections, feel less alone and more resilient on the tougher days.

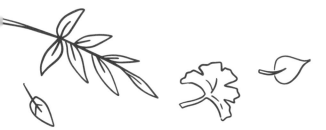

OTHER GRATITUDE PRACTICE IDEAS

- Name ten things you are grateful for in general.
- Choose a specific subject, such as individual body parts, and go into detail about what they do, how they serve you and why you value them.
- Choose a person you care about and list what it is about them you're grateful for – it's really nice to actually then write this in a letter to them. You could even send it.
- Write a gratitude list about yourself.
- Take a less structured approach – maybe it's just about making a mental note of pleasant experiences ('happy hits') as you mindfully go about your day. This could be seeing an old couple holding hands, a cute animal, a beautiful sky, a song on the radio . . . these little moments of joy that you hold onto and remember and acknowledge you felt grateful to witness.

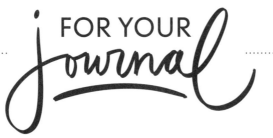

FOR YOUR journal

What would my ideal gratitude practice look like?
Do I have any resistance to gratitude? If yes, why?

How would adding in more gratitude impact my life and my wellbeing?
What are the memories or moments I can access that make my shoulders
relax and make me sigh with deep gratitude?

What am I grateful to this book for?
Who has done something special for me or has helped me?

What would it feel like to tell them? How could I tell them?
Write a letter, out loud, give them a gift?
Because I was sober, this week I . . .

WEEK 8 :
EMOTIONAL TOOLKIT
Understanding the Loneliness trigger

'Connection is the opposite of addiction.'
JOHANN HARI

We are beings who are wired for connection. According to Dacher Keltner, professor and Co-Director at The Greater Good Science Center in Berkeley, California, when we feel lonely, excluded or rejected by peers the part of our brains that is associated with pain gets activated. Scientists have also proven that loneliness and poor social contacts are associated with negative health outcomes.

Loneliness can result in using alcohol to deal with those feelings. Turning to the 'comfort' of alcohol or drugs becomes a way of coping with feeling alone, unloved, rejected or confused – it's a way to numb that pain. By making the problem/feeling go away for a little while, we avoid confronting the cause, which gives a false sense of security. It is a vicious cycle because when the drugs/alcohol are not present, all the emotions we were unable or unwilling to deal with come racing right back.

Connections and community are so important to our mental health and wellbeing. Part of the fear that many people have when they stop drinking is that it will increase their loneliness, because they are going against the social grain. The irony is that many of us sat alone on the sofa drinking or drank alone when cooking dinner. We are also told by alcohol advertising that we can't connect or feel joy without it – we need to call a halt to this and separate truth from fiction.

During the autumn months we often find it's a bit more of an effort to connect and to get out and see people. If we live on our own, we can feel this even more keenly. The micro-connections that we talked about in the spring section may dwindle as we retreat indoors and don't chat to neighbours over the fence as much, or find ourselves rushing from A to B concentrating on keeping warm rather than having a natter with a fellow dog walker. This means we need to be intentional and keep those connections topped up, to make that effort to meet friends for coffee and stay connected with each other.

Thankfully, there are scores of alcohol-free groups online now. There is honestly nothing like having a sober community to connect with and cheer you on in supporting your alcohol-free journey. This was the most significant element in early days support we could identify and is a great way to combat feelings of loneliness.

Finding an online community I could connect with and relate to was the single biggest factor in me stopping drinking. I was actually in a very lonely place, living in a new town with my husband working away, looking after the kids, isolated from my old friends and work colleagues. I turned to wine in the evenings to dull those feelings of loneliness and boredom. When I quit drinking, in the evenings I would log on to the sober forum to read, blog and chat and it was a triple-boost. It was giving me sober support, helping me understand the process I was going through and also making me feel less lonely. KATE

Loneliness was a huge trigger for me. I worked all day and then gave every last ounce of my depleted energy to my kids. My husband worked away and we live abroad in his home country, so I stared down the evening with nothing to do and no one to see. I got into the habit of keeping myself company with the TV in the background, wine in one hand and social media in the other. Part of my sober toolkit was getting a cat to keep me company – she would lie on my chest and I would feel her heartbeat. I then connected with sober forums and with their support in helping me stay sober, I started to spend the weekends really with my family rather than hungover in bed, and that helped me feel less alone. MANDY

Neurotransmitter hack – oxytocin – the connector

We can encourage feelings of safety and connection by boosting oxytocin, our love hormone. This is increased when we hug and feel intimate with others, and is also increased when we hug and feel intimate with ourselves. The brain doesn't differentiate between touch from others and touch from self, so we can create these feelings by ourselves as well as with others. Here are some natural ways to boost it:

Brain food

- Dark chocolate
- Avocados
- Salmon
- Nuts and seeds
- Mushrooms
- Eggs

Body food

- Looking after your sensory needs
- A weighted blanket
- Noise cancelling headphones
- Having a hug
- Cuddling a pet
- Cuddling a baby
- Cuddling a soft toy
- Massage and moisturizing
- Masturbating
- Holding hands (your own or others')

Soul food

- Watching feel-good films or box sets with characters we know and love
- Reaching out to people we trust either in real life or in our sober/ supportive communities
- Giving a compliment
- Acts of kindness
- Buying yourself flowers
- Self-compassion practice
- Positive affirmations
- Taking a bath

FOR YOUR *Journal*

How does loneliness show up as a trigger for me?

What can I do to make myself feel comforted?

What sober forums or sober accounts do I like?

How can I engage with them?

What steps can I take to support myself when I feel lonely?

Who is someone I can call or connect with when I need connection?

Because I was sober, this week I . . .

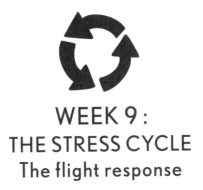

WEEK 9 :
THE STRESS CYCLE
The flight response

'Your self-love is a medicine for the Earth.'
YUNG PUEBLO

Just as birds start to head south for winter or we hurry inside to protect from autumn gusts of wind, this season lends itself to examining another aspect of our survival response – flight.

The survival response 'flight' is, as its name suggests, the urge to flee from threat or an aggressor. Just like the 'fight' response, it is fuelled by a whopping injection of adrenaline, which enables us – in the case of 'flight' – to run like the clappers. It's a really important autonomic nervous system gift, which can save our lives. It can also help us disengage from harmful conversations, assess danger and leave toxic relationships behind. As we heal, we are able to more reliably tune in to to our gut instincts and recognize when there is something we really need to flee from as opposed to our bodies triggering this response as a reaction to general life stress.

So, the survival response is ancient physiology and not an appropriate response to many modern stressors, such as utility bills or the internal critic. If we are stuck in this flight survival response mode, we live in a state of chronic stress, which has a devastating cumulative impact on our physical and mental health.

Your body undergoes a range of physiological effects when you are in the fight/flight stress response, with each body system affected. The following table is from Psychology Tools[13]:

---

13 Psychology Tools (2022). *Fight Or Flight Response*. Available at: www.psychologytools.com/resource/fight-or-flight-response

Body system	Physiological effect	Consequence
Heart	✎ Increased heart rate ✎ Dilation of coronary blood vessels	✎ Increase in blood flow ✎ Increased availability of oxygen and energy to the heart
Circulation	✎ Dilation of blood vessels serving muscles ✎ Constriction of blood vessels serving digestion	✎ Increased availability of oxygen to skeletal muscles ✎ Blood shunted to skeletal muscles and brain
Lungs	✎ Dilation of bronchi ✎ Increased respiration rate	✎ Increased availability of oxygen in blood
Liver	✎ Increased conversion of glycogen to glucose	✎ Increased availability of glucose in skeletal muscle and brain cells
Skin	✎ Skin becomes pale or flushed as blood flow is reduced	✎ Increased blood flow to muscles and away from non-essential parts of the body such as the periphery
Eyes	✎ Dilation of the pupils	✎ Allows in more light so that visual acuity is improved to scan nearby surroundings

Being stuck in this state can also lead to anxiety, obsessive or compulsive tendencies, panic and fear. It can make us restless and tap into perfectionist and workaholic tendencies. It can also impair our ability to form attachments, put down roots and get the nurture we need to be happy and healthy in our lives.

Managing 'flight', as with any of the other survival responses, is essential in maintaining sobriety. When we encounter difficulties and this response is triggered, the blood leaves our brain and we cannot make choices in line with long-term goals or approach conflict resolution in a skilful way. This is when we risk turning to old habits to cope – enter the ever-so-appealing glass of red. We need some time on our own to re-group, ground ourselves and let our system settle in the moment. There are many techniques for grounding, but a simple and effective one to remember, adapted from Therapist Aid[14], uses the five senses as a guide.

5-4-3-2-1 technique - sensory mindfulness for grounding

If you find yourself in flight mode - feeling super stressed, anxious or unable to concentrate - and fleeing is not the appropriate response, try this exercise to ground you and calm your jagged senses.

Name the following in your head or out loud, try to notice small details, and really focus in on your senses. Notice which of the senses you spend the most time on; this is an indicator of what tools you might like to add to your toolkit. For instance, you may find the sense of sight soothes you, in which case walking in beautiful scenery may be super healing for you. If you enjoy touch, then warmth, baths, blankets can all go in the toolkit. Maybe sound and music has a greater sensory impact - would noise reducing headphones change your life (like they have for us)?

	What are 5 things you can see? Look for small details such as the shadows, the reflections, the colour and depth.
	What are 4 things you can feel? Pick up an object and examine its weight, texture, and other physical qualities. Notice the sensation of clothing on your body, the sun on your skin, or the feeling of the chair you are sitting in.
	What are 3 things you can hear? What are near and distant sounds? What are sounds you no longer notice? What are natural or manmade sounds?
	What are 2 things you can smell? You may also like to take some essential oil here and take a sniff, or look around for something that has a scent, such as a flower or an unlit candle.
	What is 1 thing you can taste? Take a sip of your tea or coffee, pop in a snack or some gum and focus your attention closely on the flavours.

By doing the 5-4-3-2-1 grounding technique we anchor ourselves in the present moment and calm our nervous system.

---

14 Adapted from Therapistaid.com

To complete the whole process and return to equilibrium (from fight/flight/freeze) we also need to find ways to discharge the pent-up stress that caused the trigger in the first place. Our bodies have wanted to move, and in this case run, so naturally movement is an excellent way to do this. So, end the exercise by moving your body. You could try:

- Running
- Skipping
- Team sports (running in a pack)
- Allowing yourself to shake physically, the limbs especially
- Dynamic yoga
- Dance

If we can signal to those we love that we need some space – and they can understand this doesn't mean forever and we might need to have half an hour or a morning to ourselves – we can build trust around our needs mutually. With this communication we foster interdependence and cultivate our feelings of safety and connection. It also means that we manage our overwhelm and are not triggered to drink to try to alleviate stress or any feelings that are leading us to want to flee the situation.

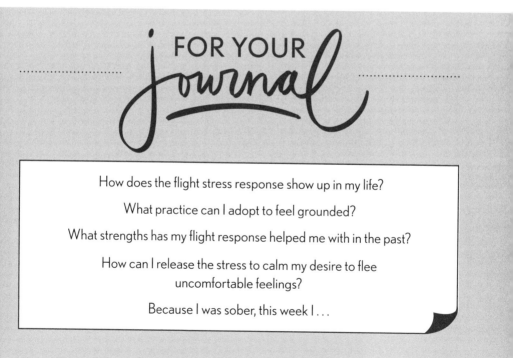

FOR YOUR Journal

How does the flight stress response show up in my life?

What practice can I adopt to feel grounded?

What strengths has my flight response helped me with in the past?

How can I release the stress to calm my desire to flee uncomfortable feelings?

Because I was sober, this week I . . .

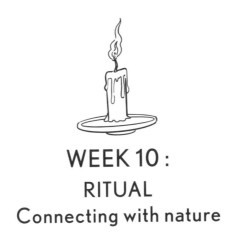

WEEK 10 :
RITUAL
Connecting with nature

'Come to the woods, for here is rest.'
JOHN MUIR

It seems ridiculous to have to point out that being in nature is good for us but in our busy, modern, linear, pavemented lives we can feel profoundly disconnected from the Great Outdoors. Walking in the woods, fields and by water we can immerse ourselves in the colours and changing temperatures of the seasons, either as a solitary practice or to be enjoyed with loved ones. Whether we like hiking up a mountain, sitting in parks with a flask of coffee or walking the dog, autumn calls to us to enjoy a bit of outside before the winter weather really kicks in. Nature can be a real gift in providing comfort and a sense of perspective of life outside of our homes, jobs and immediate problems.

Frederick Law Olmsted, the 19th-century architect of many American parks, captured the therapeutic benefits of being in the Great Outdoors. He said, 'Nature employs the mind without fatigue and yet enlivens it. Tranquilizes it and enlivens it. And thus, through the influences of the mind over body, gives the effect of refreshing rest and reinvigoration to the whole system.' Well said, sir.

How does connecting with nature help us get, stay and love being sober? By soothing ourselves in natural surroundings we can reduce triggers and cravings. If we can remove ourselves from immediate triggers and stressors and get outside and walk or run it off, this is a big old tool in our toolkits. We can also build in a regular nature practice more intentionally, not just as an emergency measure when we are about to blow our lids. In a study of 20,000 people, a team led by Dr Mathew White of the European Centre for Environment & Human Health at the University of Exeter found that people who spent two hours a week in green spaces are much more likely to identify as being physically and mentally well. Two hours minimum, he says, is the hard boundary here[15].

There is inherent wisdom and strength in Mother Nature. She carries on regardless and this can help us re-size ourselves and our problems in reference to something greater than us. In other words, she brings much needed perspective. Have you ever noticed how many of the automatic screen savers on computers are of nature scenes? Neuroscientist Stephen Kaplan showed in his labs that looking at nature pictures allowed the hard-working executive function parts of the brain to recover, compared to looking at urban landscapes[16]. Although this is not a substitute for getting outside, even looking at pictures of nature soothes us, such are our strong associations of the calming influence of nature.

The sensory and creative elements of being in nature also provide enrichment and opportunity for the state of flow, which again is soothing to the nervous systems and brings us out of those craving states. We might experiment with making jam from autumn berries and fruits or creating our own AF mixers. Making chutneys and jams also speaks to our ancestral rhythms of preparing the store cupboards for the winter months.

You only need to see kids in nature, who are natural hoarders and hedonists (but not in the three-day rave way). They delight in kicking through leaves, collecting acorns and conkers and eating blackberries. So, nature provides activities that distract us from drinking in the first place and which are inherently healing, thereby accelerating our recovery on

15 Robbins, J (2020). *Ecopsychology: How Immersion in Nature Benefits Your Health*. Available at: e360.yale.edu/features/ecopsychology-how-immersion-in-nature-benefits-your-health

16 Kaplan, S (1995). *The restorative benefits of nature: Toward an integrative framework*. Available at: www.sciencedirect.com/science/article/abs/pii/0272494495900012?via%3Dihub

many levels. And research has shown that you don't have to be in a cabin in the wilderness to reap the benefits. Local woods, water, urban parks and being in your own garden are healing, too.

I grew up in an urban environment and craved the countryside from an early age. When I went to uni in Canterbury when I was 18, it was the first time I had seen fields of yellow rapeseed and woods full of bluebells and blossom. I was captivated by the seasons. I am a truly seasonal beast and accessing nature and mindfully engaging with it is hugely important to my mental health and my creativity. KATE

I think I neglected the importance of nature in my life for a long time. It is only now in retrospect that I realize how my environment had an impact on my unhappiness. I sometimes have to force myself to get outside, but even moving my desk so it faces the window has helped my mental wellbeing. MANDY

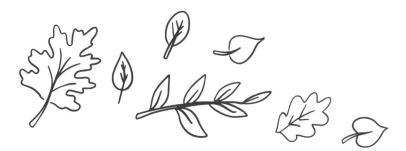

FOR YOUR *journal*

Where in nature do I get the greatest sense of relaxation?

How can I spend more time outside?

If I live in the city, how can I find ways to visit natural spaces? Are there urban green spaces I am yet to visit?

What is my favourite season?

What part does spirituality play in my life?

Where is my favourite place to visit in nature?

Because I was sober, this week I . . .

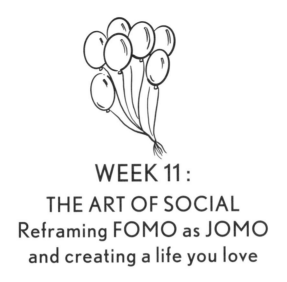

WEEK 11 :
THE ART OF SOCIAL
Reframing FOMO as JOMO
and creating a life you love

*'I am now quite cured of seeking pleasure
in society, be it country or town.'*
Catherine Earnshaw in *Wuthering Heights* by EMILY BRONTË

As we explore ways in which we want to socialize, we can rewrite the rules. The opposite of FOMO (Fear of Missing Out) is JOMO (Joy of Missing Out) which is, in our opinion, not only the best kept of secrets but in fact a superpower. FOMO is a fear-based response that was designed to keep us safe in packs. When we don't fit in and follow the herd in socio-normative ways, we fear rejection. That was all well and good when we needed to be in tight-knit groups to survive threat and attack from wolves or other tribes ... but our old physiology does not really need to fire up with the imagined threat of excommunication or death just because we see some Facebook pictures of people at the pub.

Once we understand this – and understand how marketers use it to sell us all manner of things including booze – and once we can manage that knee-jerk response with the power of the pause followed by asking ourselves what we actually want to do of an evening/holiday/weekend, we can start to be intentional about it. In other words, we can go out OR we can embrace JOMO. The choice is ours.

Before we actually get to experience JOMO we need to say 'no' to something. The power of knowing that 'no' is a full sentence isn't to be underestimated. That we don't need to tie ourselves in knots to fit in with other people's plans has been a huge learning moment for us. Saying no and being able to sit with the discomfort of others' real or imaginary disappointment takes practise for most of us. Once we have done it a few times and understand that nothing terrible happens, we learn that looking after our own needs is so much better in the long run.

So, when we are considering opting out there are a few things we need to put in place to maximize the benefits of JOMO. First, frame the JOMO as 'drawbridging.' Autumn is the perfect time to drawbridge: lighting the fire, getting cosy, watching films, cooking and taking it a bit easier. It's about balance. We don't want to disappear from civilization, but sometimes we do need to dial it down and take off the busy badge. Move away from the belief that being busy makes you worth more. When people ask you what you did at the weekend take pride in saying, 'nothing'.

We have become pretty adept at drawbridging around our own time and here are some of our big guns: on Fridays we put on Pyjama Armour and get into the Zone, which is the sofa, with a cup of tea and a blanket. If we really mean business, we have the Duvet Fortress. We delete social media apps from our phones at the weekend to ward off any random FOMO from pictures of the school mums' night out and get our chill on. We reinstate them on Sundays sometimes, so we can indulge in a bit of rewriting the language and the landscape of the morning after. Schadenfreude became Chardonnayfreude (delighting in the misery of others' hangovers) and we allow ourselves this moment. (Evil chuckle.)

Our time is precious and it is liberating to realize we can actually spend it as we wish. When you are intentionally creating a life you no longer wish to escape from, you get skillful at picking and choosing your social time. That doesn't mean you never go to the party; it's that now the choice is yours.

OUR TOP FIVE TIPS TO EMBRACE THE JOMO

- Be honest with what meets your needs. Self-care doesn't always have to be a bath with candles – it may be being creative, writing a journal, baking, singing or even therapy.
- Observe (without reacting) how it feels for you to be on your own, do nothing, please yourself, decline or cancel plans or delay responsibilities. Whatever the feelings, recognize this is an important part of your physical and emotional wellbeing.
- Pay attention to what your body is telling you. We are all affected differently by the infinite variables in our lives, whether that's the seasons, the different times of our monthly cycle or the things that trigger us.
- Consider the idea that you are enough just as you are.
- You may want a special JOMO playlist – get your pjs on, jump up and down on the bed and revel in your badassery for respecting your needs. Aretha Franklin features highly on ours: 'Sisters are Doin' It for Themselves', 'Respect' – you get the vibe.

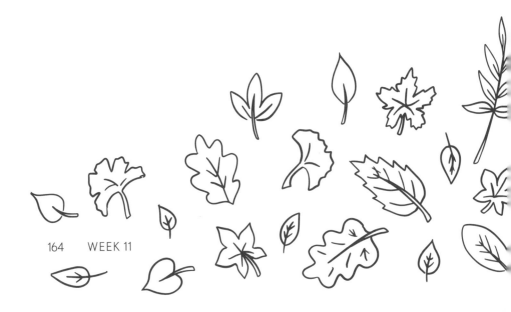

FOR YOUR *journal*

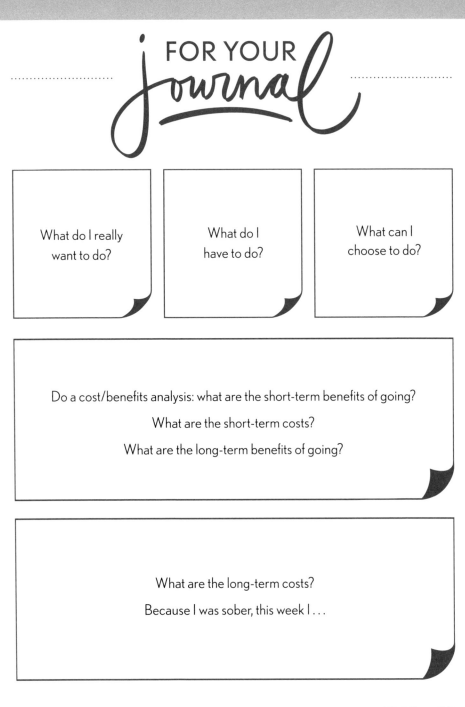

What do I really want to do?

What do I have to do?

What can I choose to do?

Do a cost/benefits analysis: what are the short-term benefits of going?

What are the short-term costs?

What are the long-term benefits of going?

What are the long-term costs?

Because I was sober, this week I . . .

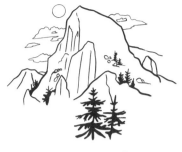

WEEK 12 :
THE SCHOOL OF LIFE
Rewriting limiting beliefs

*'Whether you think you can,
or you think you can't - you're right.'*
HENRY FORD

Beliefs are thoughts that carry a feeling of certainty about what something means. They are powerful in shaping our behaviour because, as coach Tony Robbins says, they 'create the maps that guide us toward our goals and give us the power to take action.' Most of our beliefs – both helpful and unhelpful – are generalizations about our past, based on our interpretations of painful and pleasurable experiences. They are memories that, over time, became unconscious. These memories are formed in the brain as networks of neurons that fire when stimulated by an event. The more times the network is employed, the more it fires and the stronger the memory becomes. As they say, 'neurons that fire together, wire together'.

Simply put, our limiting beliefs can cause us to miss out and our empowering beliefs can help us succeed. An example of this could be believing you won't get the job before you even walk into the interview – this is a pretty negative starting point and may well influence how you act and lessen your chances. On the other hand, believing you can get the job is likely to give you a more positive demeanor from the outset.

We want to tread carefully here, because it can be toxically positive to pretend it's all in the mind. Life is not a level playing field and sometimes terrible things happen and it's important we recognize this. However, if we work with the internal and external messages we received about ourselves, we can move out of unconscious reaction and start to move to a more positive proactive place.

If our beliefs change, the way we act and/or feel will change, too. Slowly, by making them conscious, challenging them, trying new things and collecting new evidence, we may surprise ourselves and build a new sense of who we are and what we can do. We got to rewrite our beliefs that we needed alcohol to de-stress and enjoy ourselves and have become two women who love being sober. Sobriety gave us the opportunity to rewrite our opinions of ourselves, changing from feeling fearful, flakey, ashamed and sad to courageous, resilient, proud and excited about life. Change is possible!

FOR YOUR *Journal*

We're going to suggest something different for your journaling this week and delve a little deeper to help you challenge limiting beliefs with the following seven steps, adapted from the American Writers & Artists Institute. Make a list of any negative self-beliefs you may hold and then challenge one at a time.

SAMPLE BELIEF: I can't give up booze for good as I will never be able to enjoy a party sober.

Step #1 – Question the belief

Ask yourself the following three questions:

- Do I really know that this is true? (I don't know, I haven't done it for a while.)
- Have I experienced this myself enough times to be confident that it is true? (It's been true for a while but I remember enjoying parties as a kid.)
- Do I really know that this belief is true, without a shred of doubt? (Hmmm . . . I might have to give it a go to see. . . .)

These are powerful questions when answered honestly. Do not underestimate or skip this step. It is vital to your ability to create a new life without limits.

Step #2 – Dig deeper

Where did you come up with this belief? (It's been like this for a long time.)
Your beliefs should come from your own personal experiences and from the advice of experts. (Experts would probably say I actually can enjoy a party and if I can't then something definitely needs to change.)

Step #3 – Dethrone the old belief

Simply state to yourself, 'I choose not to believe this anymore. It's not true.' Now imagine, vividly and in writing, how much your life would change if you didn't have this belief in your life. (Wafting around a party, belly laughing with besties and leaving looking gorgeous, sleeping like a baby and waking up hangover free.)

Step #4 – Create a new belief that serves you

This will be the opposite of the limiting belief, or at least something along those lines. Create a belief that will improve your life and support your ability to take action to make your life better. Use a mantra, such as 'I am enjoying a party sober and leaving when I have had enough.' Then, go and road-test it.

Step #5 – Monitor your progress

After the event, check yourself. How do you feel about your new belief? How do you feel about your old belief? Check your gut; it's a direct link to your subconscious. Ask yourself, 'Is my behaviour changing? Do I have any new evidence?'

Step #6 – Repeat

Go back to your list of limiting beliefs. Keep working on them and continue to add new items as and when they arise.

Step #7 – Repeat the repeat

Continue regularly examining your life for limiting beliefs and eliminating them. It's like pulling weeds. No matter what you do, some weeds always pop up over time. Simply recognize them and get rid of them. With regular practice this becomes easier.

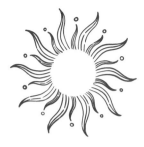

WEEK 13 :
TOOLS FOR GREATER REFLECTION
Self-compassion

'Remember, you have been criticizing yourself for years and it hasn't worked. Try approving of yourself and see what happens.'
LOUISE L HAY

As we start to turn inward in the autumn months, we come face to face with ourselves. Things we may have been ignoring successfully by keeping busy and distracted in the summer months may rear their ugly heads and start jostling for our attention. Self-compassion is the care and nurturing we offer ourselves when we come to meet ourselves as we are, warts and all, when we make mistakes, embarrass ourselves, or come short of a goal we were hoping to achieve. It is the acknowledgment of our pain, and the rejection of the notion that we should just tough it out.

Gah! Self-compassion is quite possibly the hardest and yet most rewarding and fruitful gift we have to give ourselves in our lives. When is it we start showing up with our best interests at heart? When will we let go and forgive ourselves for the mistakes we have made? When will we treat ourselves with compassion when we perceive we have failed, are inadequate or are struggling?

Self-compassion is a profound practice of self-love. When you can stop hating on yourself for the past, recognize the disconnect and be able to self-parent in order to live with the intention of no self-harm, you won't put a poison like alcohol in your precious self anymore. It's cheesy but you are worth it and you have to know you are!

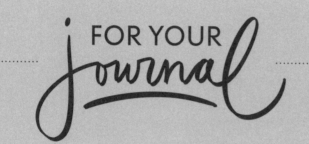

FOR YOUR Journal

How can I strengthen my relationship with myself on a regular basis?

What kind words can I tell myself right now?

What am I proud of achieving?

What am I sorry that happened to me?

How can I provide myself comfort?

Because I was sober, this week I . . .

AUTUMN EQUINOX
Ritual and reflection

Autumn Equinox is traditionally the time of the final harvest. When people lived more closely connected to the Earth this was the time of year they'd celebrate the abundance of summer. The extremes of summer and winter are once again touched by a transition point and we have another equinox when the balance of light and dark is equal. The sense of this season is gathering what we have sown and worked hard for on our sober journey, reflecting on our own personal sober harvests, celebrating and at the same time preparing for leaner, darker months.

Nature releases what's no longer needed in line with the Panarchic theory and the equinox can be seen as an opportunity to audit or edit our lives. This moment to pause and take stock can help us to reflect on what is working and what needs a tweak. Widening the aperture to look at areas such as work/life balance, rest/play balance, social/alone-time balance can help us to make adjustments. When these areas are well balanced, it's like having a broad base that allows us to maintain greater emotional equilibrium which, in turn, makes us more resilient and less likely to get knocked off balance and reach for the wine.

We know that transitions can be tricky and the transition to winter can definitely feel like a bumpy descent, an airplane coming in to land. As the damp creeps in and we feel that pull to go inward, note what comes up. Is it a relief or a feeling of sadness as we head into winter and our serotonin levels can drop with the lack of light? Is it a bit of both? Choose something from your growing toolkit to meet that need and sustain you. If we have prepped the route, know the conditions and are skilled pilots, it will make for a smoother landing. So, in this moment let's pause and reflect on our internal weather and check in with our self-care controls so we can bring ourselves down to earth for the winter months without a bump.

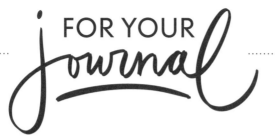
FOR YOUR
Journal

What were my autumn wins?
What challenges did I overcome this autumn?
What would I like to rewrite?

What am I proud of?
What's not working anymore for me?
What feels tired and needs a rest?

What do I need to add in and let go of to replenish and sustain my
sobriety at this point in the year?
How will I reward myself?

In what areas of my life do I feel really well-balanced?
Where do I feel like I am rockin' it?
Because I was sober, this week I . . .

Winter

'Winter, a lingering season, is a time to gather golden moments, embark upon a sentimental journey, and enjoy every idle hour.'
JOHN BOSSWELL

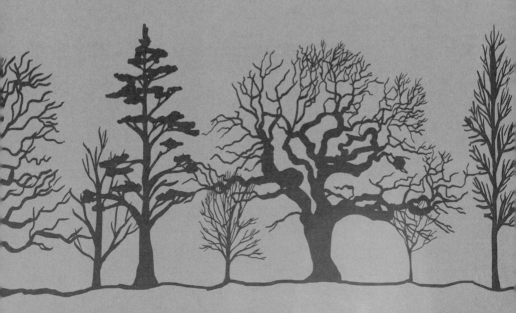

HARNESSING THE POWER OF THE GIFTS OF WINTER TO REST

As winter approaches, we enter the REST phase of the R4 Balance cycle, which chimes with the winter phase of the Panarchic theory (the cyclical pattern we see in the seasons) as we allow stillness and space to consolidate the learning from the previous cycles of growth, conservation and release and begin the process of reorganization and contemplation for our next cycle of growth in spring. The darkness and cold of this season invite us to huddle and feast, wrap up and snuggle down, and find a woman cave in which to spend some time reflecting. We are encouraged by the wisdom of nature to take a more passive role, to rest as much as we can, to sleep, to hibernate, to adjust our diet to warming soups and stews, and to attend to the lighting in our homes to counteract the darkness outside.

Winter is magical with its fires, crisp mornings and twinkling fairy lights. In the Northern Hemisphere, we have the often-boozy festivals of Christmas and New Year (in the Southern Hemisphere, of course, these fall in the heady, hectic summer) and we need to plan for these, organizing and utilizing a next-level toolkit, which we will explore in this section. Even if you don't celebrate Christmas, the booze advertising machine is heavy on the 'you can't connect without alcohol' message so it's really useful to recognize this and plan accordingly.

Reflection, planning, taking stuff off the to-do lists and keeping an eye on expectations is all a must. We can then fill our sober stockings with all the things we need and deserve as we cultivate reflection and hope in our hearts and with our loved ones throughout the dark months.

In winter, rest is not only important to nourish and restore our bodies but also our projects. Periods of retreat and rest are vital for reaching our long-term goals. This is the ebb to the flow, our opportunity to refuel, restock and replenish. Winter is nature's way of preparing for the renewal of spring. In our sobriety, no matter what happens, we never return to exactly the same point as before, even if it may feel like it if we have had a slip up and had a period of drinking that interrupted our growth cycle. Like the fields lying dormant to allow for spring crops, there will be some tiny seed of new learning or expanded awareness growing within us.

Return to this section whenever you need to rest, contemplate and reorganize in order to move forward.

REASONS TO BE CHEERFUL IN WINTER

Open fires, chilly mornings, mittens, crunchy walks in the fields, holly, ice skating, winter solstice, candles, bobble hats, frost, hot chocolate, clementines, chai tea, AF mulled wine, soups, fairy lights, beautiful sunrises and sunsets.

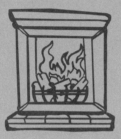 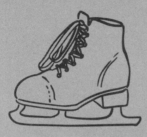 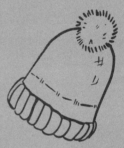

FOR YOUR JOURNAL

How do I want to feel this winter?

What matters to me the most this season?

When do I feel my most happy/calm/joyful?

What would I like to create or nurture in my life this season?

What elements make winter special for me?

What fears would I like to release this winter?

Because I was sober, this week I . . .

WEEK 1:
YOUR SEASONAL PLANNER

'The secret of getting ahead is getting started.'
AGATHA CHRISTIE

Let's have a look at the overview of your winter. As with every season, we are designing our life map according to the natural features and lay of the land and planning our route to better prepare for our journey. What is impactful about this season for you? What holidays or extra family commitments do you have coming up? What challenges might they bring? How can you take things off the list to focus on rest? What fun things have you got to look forward to? What commitments do you resent that need to be rethought? How can you delegate? What are you looking forward to?

Fill in your simple planner to note your intentions for specific dates and some questions for deeper reflection as you rest in winter!

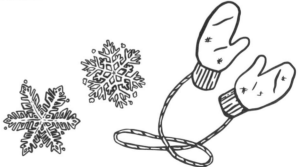

WINTER
Planner

Month 1

Month 2

Month 3

Hobbies to try

....

....

....

Key dates

Possible Triggers

Strategy ....

Movement ....

Self-care ....

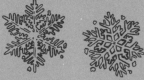

HOW TO USE YOUR PLANNER FOR WINTER

If this is your first sober winter how can you get cosy in this delicious season? Adjust your self-care to suit the winter energy. Do you feel like changing up your exercise? Perhaps getting some AF drinks for social occasions and changing your wardrobe to suit the shift in seasons? Plan in plenty of time to focus on your own self-care in this season, which is often heavily focused on meeting the needs of others. Plan in some winter fun.

Check in with your feelings about this time of year. As with the other seasons, we challenge you to:

- Try a new alcohol-free drink
- Read a new book
- Do a new hobby or activity that you have always wanted to try
- Say no to something you don't want to do
- Add in some movement
- Add in some self-care

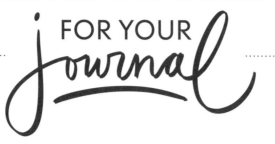

FOR YOUR Journal

What associations do I have with these major dates coming up?
How confident on a scale of 1 to 10 do I feel about managing this period alcohol free?
Which activities do I want to opt out of this year?
What key dates have I identified that are important to me?

How do they normally relate to drinking alcohol?
What new rituals can I introduce?
Are there certain dates I need to plan around because of alcohol?
What will I do?

What do I need to do to increase my confidence level by 1 point?
(Have a friend there, opt out, drive, journal more, get a coach?)
What might I do instead?
What might I drink instead?

What can I plan in instead?
Because I was sober, this week I . . .
What is your confidence level now from 1 to 10? Hopefully it will have improved.
If not, go back and see if you can generate more options.

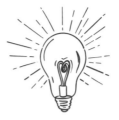

WEEK 2:
SETTING YOUR INTENTION
The power of the pause and how to
cultivate patience

'Patience is bitter, but its fruit is sweet.'
JEAN-JACQUES ROUSSEAU

Winter is a season that demands we be patient. It reminds us that we must wait for the light, for new shoots to appear and for new cycles of growth. We may be used to rushing but the seasons have their own timings. We also need to be patient with ourselves, of course. Changing our habits takes perseverance, so we need to keep momentum by regularly celebrating our progress, giving ourselves high fives and noticing the little things. This may sound simple but it really does help to cultivate patience for the bigger shifts and rewards we are waiting for on this sober journey, such as feeling free from alcohol and not wanting alcohol. So, remind yourself, you are doing amazingly, you are worth it and you have NO idea how good you are going to feel this time next year. Trust the path and keep going. Do less, let time do more.

The ability to defer gratification is part of our brain's 'executive function' skill set, which governs memory, mental flexibility and self-control. This area of the brain normally develops as we get older – witness the toddler having a meltdown in the supermarket because he can't have sweets. As we grow up, the executive function skill set becomes more developed, reaching maturity in our 20s. However, this part of the brain is impacted by all sorts of challenges: trauma, developmental issues, neurodiversity, poverty, genetics and by using substances like alcohol.

There is no way round developing the ability to ride out cravings if we are to beat the Wine Witch. We need to practise, repeatedly, the power of the pause. It is THE sober masterclass because when we are patient, when we press the HALT button instead of the F*** It button and stop and step back for a moment, we allow our logical brains time to come back online, see the bigger picture and create rather than react. We reach for our sober toolkits instead of for that bottle of vino. This, in a nutshell, is the secret of success.

Cultivating patience is quite simple in theory. It's like building a muscle through reps. We can develop the skill by learning to make ourselves wait and building the capacity to tolerate the feeling of wanting. You could try with something like a cup of tea. If you want a cup of tea, make yourself wait five minutes. If we try with little habits like this that have less of an addictive charge it can build resilience overall, which will indirectly help us tolerate cravings.

Secondly, we need to reduce stress generally. If we are stressed and in fight/flight mode we will be highly reactive, and no good decisions are made when in this state. Using the self-care tools discussed in this book – such as walks in nature, connection, movement and mindfulness practice – we will also help build the patience muscle because we are routinely practising self-care and stress management. The calmer we are, the more patient we are.

When we build the patience muscle it directly helps us manage our cravings. If we are crying out for that glass of wine at 5pm but we are patient with ourselves and slow ourselves down with a practice of flow (playing Tetris, chopping vegetables, colouring, doing a puzzle) and wait, we see that trigger and craving subside. This builds confidence because we now have evidence that we can get through it.

As newly sober people we will tend to be more at the reactive end of the patience spectrum and will be faced with cravings. We need to work at cultivating the skill of patience and wherever we are on our sober journeys we need to carry on practising it as an ongoing inoculation against our (completely human) addictive, impatient tendencies.

"Trust the path and keep going.
Do less, let time do more."

FOR YOUR *journal*

How easy is it for me to wait for things?

What can I do when I have a compulsive urge to react?

What is the best way for me to distract myself for 15 mins?

What is my go-to tool to calm myself down?

Are there certain situations where I feel very impatient?

How can I mark my daily successes and notice the little things? Because I was sober, this week I . . .

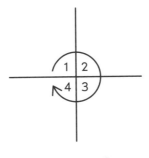

WEEK 3 :
CYCLES AND SOBRIETY
The 7 Cs of resilience

'Do not judge me by my success, judge me by how many times I fell down and got back up again.'
NELSON MANDELA

One of the beautiful outcomes of sober living is increased resilience, that super power of being able to bounce back from the stuff life throws at us, like Elastigirl. Although being alcohol-free is not the panacea to solve all of life's problems, it certainly does deal with many of them and we no longer have all of the misery that alcohol brings all by itself. We are hangover-free, more regulated, have more money, energy and peace of mind – not to mention glowing skin, better hair and brighter eyes. All this, simply because we have stepped off the drinking merry-go-round, fuelled as it is by shame, regret and cravings. Turning up day in day out to your life and meeting challenges and joys head on means you are basically a warrior goddess. You are She-Ra.

Winter is a perfect season to reflect on your resilience, see it, feel it, acknowledge it, applaud it and nurture it. This, in turn, will feed it all the more.

American pediatrician and development expert, Dr Kenneth Ginsburg, suggests seven components that make up resilience, and we have adapted these to apply them to your sobriety.

THE 7 Cs OF SOBER RESILIENCE

1. Competence

This is the ability to know how to handle stressful situations effectively. It requires having the skills to face challenges, and having had the opportunity to practise using these skills. As you witness yourself doing what you say you will (clocking up your sober days) you notice and reinforce your competence.

2. Confidence

This is the belief in one's own abilities and it is rooted in competence. We gain confidence by being able to demonstrate we are competent in real situations. Seeing is believing, and conquering situations sober hugely increases your confidence in your ability to live a life free from alcohol.

3. Connection

When we have close ties to friends, family and community groups we are more likely to have a stronger sense of security, common values and belonging, and we are less likely to seek out destructive behaviours. By joining a sober community we can feel robust and grounded. We had a common problem and now share the common value that sobriety is important to us. When our resilience is low, others can hold the ground for us. As the She Recovers motto so rightly says, 'together we are stronger'.

4. Character

This is about having a strong sense of self-worth and confidence. We demonstrate a caring attitude toward others, have boundaries and live by our values. We have a strong sense of right and wrong and are prepared to make wise choices and contribute to the world. One of the awesome things about being sober is you REALLY get to know yourself. You rediscover loves, hates, preferences, whims, foibles, dreams – all the things that make you so beautifully unique. We stop people-pleasing and show up authentically and with purpose, and we look after ourselves with healthy boundaries.

5. Contribution

When we can experience personally contributing to the world, we learn the powerful lesson that the world is a better place because we are in it. Hearing the appreciation when we contribute increases our willingness to take actions and make choices that improve the world, enhancing our own competence, character and sense of connection. Being seen by sober people and, in turn, perhaps being an example or a support for someone else who is questioning their drinking makes you feel badass.

6. Coping

This is about having a wide repertoire of coping skills, and being able to cope more effectively and be better prepared to overcome life's challenges. Hello sober toolkit. We have many resources and this keeps growing as we progress to authentically help soothe, calm, invigorate and grow equal to life's challenges. WE KNOW WE GOT THIS!

7. Control

When we realize we have control over our decisions and actions, we are more likely to know how to make choices in a way that helps us to bounce back from life's challenges. In the words of the Serenity Prayer, 'Grant me the serenity to accept the things I cannot change, the courage to change the things I can, and the wisdom to know the difference.'

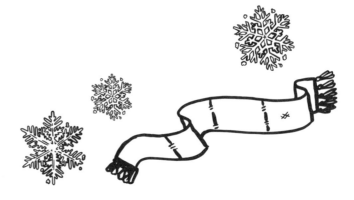

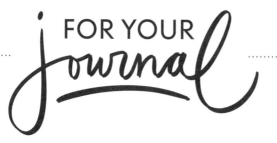
FOR YOUR
journal

How resilient do I feel at the moment?
When I have had periods of not drinking, when did I falter?
Which of the 7 Cs do I feel is my strongest?

Which of the 7 Cs do I think I need to nurture?
Which practices build resilience for me?
What life events can I foresee where my decision to be
alcohol-free might be challenged?

What might I do to strengthen my resilience if that were to happen?
Because I was sober, this week I . . .

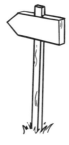

WEEK 4:
CULTIVATING SOBER SPACE
Acceptance

*'Life is a series of natural and spontaneous changes.
Don't resist them; that only creates sorrow. Let reality be reality.
Let things flow naturally forward in whatever way they like.'*
LAO TZU

Acceptance is so important on our sober journey. We are in the process of accepting that we are ending our relationship with alcohol. We need to accept that what we're seeking (being care-free drinkers) has gone, accept we have done things we weren't proud of, accept that we have, at times, put ourselves at risk or shouted at our kids when we were hungover. In the work of acceptance there has to be honesty, compassion for others and compassion for ourselves.

Acceptance isn't about agreeing with something or necessarily liking it – it's about choosing grace over drama, peace over chaos, and the willingness to give up suffering over something we cannot control. This might be mistakes we made in the past around our ability to control alcohol. It's exhausting to fight reality and, on top of that, it doesn't work; it only holds us back and keeps us stuck in old patterns, beliefs and unhealthy situations.

We spent most of our lives feeling ashamed, guilty and not good enough, and our drinking was a way to escape. We were caught up in old stories and to really heal we had to let those stories go. Perhaps there were some amends to make, but there was also a need for recognition of how we had been mistreated or/and wronged, by ourselves, by society and by alcohol itself. We weren't the problem, alcohol was.

At Love Sober we strove to create a model of ending our relationship with alcohol from an empowered place. We have a couple of Love Sober mantras we cling to: 'What happened, happened', and 'It is what it is'. You can hear us muttering these fairly often, as well as, 'I am perfectly imperfect and that's enough'. The traditional requirement of Alcoholics Anonymous to list our character defects, check our egos and 'admit' we were 'powerless over alcohol' felt counterproductive to us as women and entirely the wrong approach to healing the hurts and stress that had led us to getting ourselves mixed up with alcohol in the first place. So, rather than admitting we were 'flawed' and 'powerless', we accepted that alcohol was damaging us, we accepted that alcohol marketing was BS and we healed from a place of self-care and self-love, rather than shame.

However, getting to that empowered, fire-in-your-belly, 'F*** you, alcohol!' place does take time. Something that isn't often talked about with positive sobriety models is that, for some, there is a sense of loss and grieving for alcohol and the times that you had that may have been good. This is part of the sober journey and it's perfectly OK to feel sad about saying goodbye to your old friend vino, as long as you don't get stuck there.

The process we follow in getting, staying and learning to love sober follows that of the Kübler-Ross Change Curve (also known as the 5 Stages of Grief). It is a model consisting of the various levels or stages of emotions experienced by a person who is soon going to approach death or has lost a loved one. This model was introduced by and is named after Elisabeth Kübler-Ross in her 1969 book *On Death and Dying*. We realized that with all change comes a kind of grieving – whether it be the end of a relationship or a child leaving home, perhaps – and the same goes for breaking up with booze.

At first there is denial: we tell ourselves, 'Surely I am not that bad? Everyone drinks like me.' Next comes frustration and depression when we realize change has been thrust upon us and something has to give. 'Why me?' we cry. After this comes the acceptance that there is a line that has been crossed with alcohol and we can never go back. As William Porter says in his book Alcohol Explained, 'When it's soured, it's soured.' Once we accept that we will never be happy-go-lucky drinkers and that, at best, we will always be trying hard to control alcohol and, at worst, we will develop severe dependency to it, we can start to experiment with what a life beyond the shackles of alcohol might look like. We generate new options and look forward rather than back. Finally, we make the decision to change and integrate this new way of being into who we are.

With acceptance we understand that we did the best we could at the time with what we had. We cannot change the past. What we can do is put our best foot forward and, in choosing sobriety, we do the next right thing and then the next, without our judgement being clouded by booze, which is a powerful antidote to shame. The rest simply has to be good enough.

The Kübler-Ross Change Curve

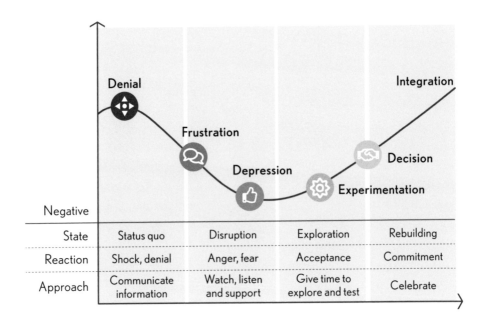

	State	Status quo	Disruption	Exploration	Rebuilding
	Reaction	Shock, denial	Anger, fear	Acceptance	Commitment
	Approach	Communicate information	Watch, listen and support	Give time to explore and test	Celebrate

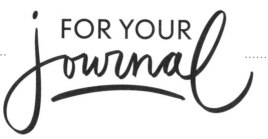

FOR YOUR journal

Where do I see myself on the change curve? What do I need right now?

List all the things that I feel guilty or ashamed about in the past in relation to drinking and ask, would I have done those things if I were sober?

Would I like to make amends to anyone? Say sorry for something?

What past stories am I holding on to that are self-harming and stopping me moving forward?

What is in my control to change now?

How can I be my best friend and let things go?

What have I done well?

When I let the inner critic speak, how is it wrong?

If I could tell my younger self something, what would I say?

Because I was sober, this week I . . .

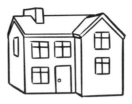

WEEK 5:
BOSSING YOUR ENVIRONMENT
Sacred space and woman caves

*'Having a safe space to imagine and dream and (re)invent
yourself is the first step to being happy and successful,
whatever road you choose to pursue.'*
ASHLEY BRYAN

In our overpopulated world, with our busy lives and ever-encroaching tech, places of solitude are hard to come by. Newsflash! Distractions will not remove themselves and information overload does not manage itself. Therefore, it is our responsibility to intentionally and mindfully slow down and create extra space if we want to take charge of reactions and triggers around alcohol. We see the woman cave as more than just a room – it's an actual physical sacred space in which we can retreat, restore and regain equilibrium away from the constant hum of noise.

We women, despite having so much weight on our shoulders, are rarely given (or rarely give ourselves) permission to take space. We run ourselves ragged taking care of the kids and other loved ones and tend to worry about every small detail. If you're a caregiver, woman or not, you deserve a 'cave' – a place that you can escape to in order to cultivate calmness, creativity and relaxation.

Many of us who become alcohol-free, at some point realize we have been using alcohol in part to claim space for ourselves. We used it to numb sensory overload, to calm social anxiety – like the discomfort of being in loud, smelly, crowded bars – and as a temporary way to make it go quiet in our own homes. So, if a woman cave seems frivolous or indulgent, reframe it right now as an act of survival. If an animal is stressed or overwhelmed it will find somewhere to hide. We need that 'luxury', too.

Sacred spaces have been used for ritual, celebration and reflection for eons, with tools and symbols to focus minds and intentions. Witches and Wiccans cast circles; priests lay the altars. These are actually no different from turning off your phone and sitting on the patio to mindfully drink some tea and do a bit of journaling. They are simply tools and practices to signal some time that is separate from the hustle of life – a boundary. Remember, we are in the process of reclaiming space and calling on our wisest selves to live intentionally here. We can't do this if we can't escape dirty washing and constant demands from time to time.

Obviously, however much we may want to manifest a spa/hammam with silks, candles, a roll top bath and plinky-plonky music while being fed grapes by firemen (sorry, did we take that too far?) this may not be feasible. However, spotting the triggers and planting the idea that you deserve to take some time out can be the starting point for a calmer you.

In our modern lives, our sacred space could be a yoga mat, or a café where we go to work with our noise-reducing headphones and listen to 80s power ballads. (No? Just us then?)

Perhaps your woman cave is a sunny spot outside, a favourite walk, a place in the park with a particular view. Whatever it may be, it's a place where you can be away from people, to focus on you. It's somewhere you can use as an anchor in times of stress, and a place to make the world go a bit quiet.

When the world goes quiet, we can process life, identify our needs and reconnect with what's important to us. We can, when we shut out the noise for long enough, begin to hear the whispers of self, of wishes and of those things that are important to us. Not the to-dos, not the shoulds but those heart-whispers of self.

KATE'S WOMAN CAVE: My office. It has yoga stuff, a desk, books, candles, devotional things, and gifts people have given me, as well as journals and a mala bracelet-making kit, my computer and essential oils. I fought tooth and nail for it. My husband moved in there during lockdown. Gradually, without saying a word, over a few weeks I removed his things and put mine back in, like a game of Risk, and in the end, he moved out downstairs to work. YAS, QUEEN! (Does victory dance.)

MANDY'S WOMAN CAVE: My bathroom. Candles and a bath (luckily now my kids are older they won't bother me in there!). I have some speakers to listen to tunes, podcasts or meditations, some comforting books, essential oils, Epsom salts and the door is CLOSED.

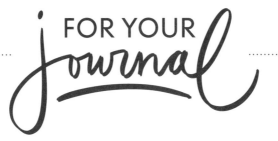

FOR YOUR
journal

What do I need to do to create space for myself?

Where is the place in my house where I feel calmest?

What would be one thing I could add to create some sparkle
and magic in my home?

How can I create boundaries with those I live with to protect my space?

What does space mean to me?

Because I was sober, this week I . . .

WEEK 6 :
RESEARCHING OUR RESOURCES
Storytelling and community

'Shame dies when stories are told in safe spaces.'
ANN VOSKAMP

Winter's darkness provides opportunities to reflect and create new narratives about how we would like things to change, as we take a moment to pause and reflect and also to think about the start of another cycle of the seasons. The opposite of giddy, extroverted summer, it calls us to be inside and pulls our gaze closer and inside ourselves.

Storytelling is a fundamental part of being human. Before the written word, oral traditions allowed us to pass down wisdom through generations, sharing our evolutions, struggles and triumphs. In her book *If Women Rose Rooted* Dr Sharon Blackie discusses how women's stories, heroines and archetypes became watered down once the word was committed to page by monks (men). Now that we can write, and have access to the internet and social media, we have never had such an opportunity to tell our stories and be heard.

The simple act of writing down our own drinking story can be one of the most transformative practices. When we are deep in the day-to-day of our lives we lack perspective, like focusing in closely on stitches in a handmade tapestry. The act of stepping back and viewing our timeline, major events and significant players can be like stepping back and assessing our handiwork, and allows us greater opportunity to decide which next stitches to make. We can finally take stock of our 'herstory' and make sense of how we got to where we are now.

Our story does not need to be *Anna Karenina*. We can write it for the hell of it, publish it, burn it. It's ours. And just the act of the hand moving across the page in a stream of consciousness is therapeutic, it doesn't have to be good. We can tell our stories through Instagram posts, blogs, diaries, poetry and photography to name just a few. We can use storytelling as a private reflective practice and as a way to connect with others. Perhaps we start by journaling and, as we grow in confidence, start a blog or become more engaged on online forums. Perhaps we start a podcast? We have a good friend Nancy (@sober_loving_radical) who tells her sober story through dancing and music on TikTok.

As we have said before, when we engage our creative mind (the right side) it helps our healing and transformation. Storytelling allows us to see ourselves as part of a bigger picture of a greater story and that helps us feel less alone. Storytelling breaks down stigma and shame, it gives us context. We can rewrite our story and see it through the eyes of someone else – how does it change when we see it from a different perspective? Do we feel more compassion? Are we able to access greater wisdom or perspective?

When we do feel ready to share our stories in safe spaces, we are seen, we connect and we can heal as we are reminded that, in hearing others' stories, we are more alike than not and we all have joys and sorrows. Storytelling connects us to our common humanity, especially when we are surrounded by people who get it, and have travelled the same path. We can take a big sigh of relief knowing that things will now get easier.

We encourage you to tell your story in some way to someone. This could be anonymously on a sober site such as Soberistas, it could be in a small community such as ours at Love Sober, or it could be to someone close to you or a doctor, therapist or coach. Perhaps you want to write it first, or say it out loud, but when you can, let someone in and let them know the real you; that is when you will finally draw a line under the secrets that have been keeping you stuck.

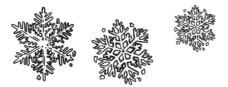

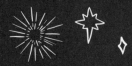

"Storytelling breaks down
stigma and shame,
it gives us context."

FOR YOUR *Journal*

What is the story I would like to tell my younger self of how I changed my life for the better?

If a fictional character or cartoon could play me in my life story, who would it be and why?

When I think about alcohol as an evil character, who is it? What do they look like?

What superpower do I possess to keep me on my alcohol-free path?

Which sober people are my inspirations?

What community would I like to be a part of?

Because I was sober, this week I . . .

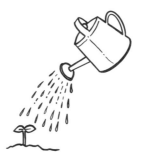

WEEK 7 :
FOSTERING POSITIVE GROWTH
Self-leadership

*'Leadership and learning are
indispensable to each other.'*
JOHN F KENNEDY

Resting and reorganizing in winter is about getting stronger. We are building sober muscle and sober skill, and learning the essential art of self-leadership. For many years, so many of us have looked for confirmation of our worth from outside. In sobriety, we get to clear away the noise of alcohol and have the opportunity to ask ourselves questions like: What do I really like? What do I really want? What do I really need? And this can feel scary as f***.

In Tara Mohr's brilliant book *Playing Big* she writes about a process of 'unhooking from praise and criticism', where she discusses how we are conditioned to measure our self-worth by how well we perform in the eyes of others, rather than how we actually feel about ourselves. We get caught up in perfectionism and people-pleasing and lose ourselves in the process. In our experience, drinking was an extension of this disconnect and tendency to outsource confidence and self-belief to alcohol, which in turn destroyed it.

Because women often feel a duty to care for others, we often want to be kind, and to be experienced as kind, which is the positive side of our relationship focus. The negative side is that we compromise a sense of self due to our fear of not belonging. We silence ourselves so as not to rock the boat which, in turn, leaves us disconnected from what really matters to us. We tend to be empathic and pick up on the emotional reactions of others. We become chameleon-like in our attempts to meet everyone's needs, notice non-verbal cues and adapt ourselves. This can be a strength, but can be exhausting.

We also have a history of survival through likeability and social influence. In the past, women survived by being nice and being passive; we didn't have economic freedom or the physical strength to fight. 'Good-girl conditioning' and being judged on our looks meant we learned that praise was equal to love. We often never feel good enough or qualified enough if we are not in high-performance mode and this holds us back from doing what we really desire and answering our own needs.

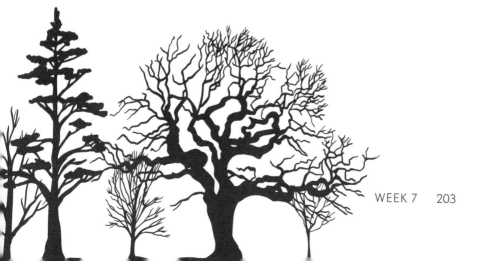

How can we unhook from praise and criticism as markers of our worth? In *Playing Big*, Tara suggests the following, which we heartily endorse:

Remember feedback doesn't always tell you about you; it tells you about the person giving the feedback.

Often, especially around our decision to stop drinking, some people can become defensive, rude or mocking. What does that tell you about their insecurity around their drinking? If they praise you when you drink, is it for your benefit or theirs?

Incorporate feedback that's strategically useful, and let the rest go.

A lot of us go into crisis mode when receiving any feedback – we need to slow down and ask ourselves, what of this works for me? What information will help me grow? What of this is aligned with my values? Leave the rest.

Women who play big get criticized. Period.

Some people are not going to like your strength, new-found edges and boundaries, but that doesn't mean you're wrong to change. It just means people will need time to adjust or they don't really have your back after all.

Criticism hurts when it mirrors what we believe about ourselves.

Ouch Tara, OUCH! When you really think about it, not all criticism hurts the same – sometimes we brush it off and sometimes we feel like the world will end ... but why? It's because deep down what they have said is what we believe or fear about ourselves. We can use this knowledge to take back power and challenge those negative feelings we have about ourselves and look for evidence that it isn't true ... even if it may have been true in the past. Today you own your own destiny and today you can shape your future.

Ask, what's more important to me than praise?

This one is SO helpful in your sobriety, because ultimately not harming yourself IS more important than praise. No one else is in your life, in your shoes, and no one else's experience matters. Know this if you are reading this book: YOU are worth more than being convenient for other people.

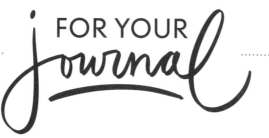

FOR YOUR Journal

What would I need to feel confident to take leadership in my own life?
What can I do to protect myself in relationships and not slip into martyrdom?

What can help me to hear my own wants, needs and boundaries
amongst the noise of other people's needs?

What is more important to me than praise?
If I have/did have a daughter how would I like her to journey through the world?

What other qualities would I like people to see in me apart from being nice?
Because I was sober, this week I . . .

WEEK 8 :
EMOTIONAL TOOLKIT
Understanding the Tiredness trigger

'I am so tired even my tiredness is tired.'
ANON

Tiredness is an almost universal booze trigger for women. We so often feel bone-tired, don't we? We go on the hunt for a magic solution in the form of vitamins and minerals, pills and potions, while never getting enough time and rest, which are the true healers.

Our bodies love routines and rhythms and having a good evening routine is an important foundation for the transition to rest and sleep. Although alcohol can make us fall asleep, the dysregulation of blood sugar it causes throughout the night means, for many of us, 3am anxiety, heart palpitations and insomnia.

We often drink when we feel tired because it gives us temporary fuel, a false boost of energy and masks the feelings of being tired. In turn, this makes us more tired, dehydrated and lethargic and often robs us of a good night's sleep. This see-saw of dysregulation means we have limited capacity to deal with stress and are increasingly vulnerable to the calls of the Wine Witch. We need to build in regular rest periods for ourselves and to do this intentionally because no one is going to tell us to take a day off or leave the washing till later.

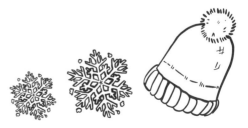

5 TOOLS TO COMBAT TIREDNESS

There IS such a thing as a free lunch

Fuel yourself with morning and afternoon healthy snacks like fruit, nuts or yoghurt. Take an actual lunch break at lunchtime and make sure you eat around the middle of your day. Get some fresh air and move around to get the oxygen pumping round the body to help release stress.

Mini breaks vs mini dramas

Taking mini breaks throughout the day helps build capacity and regulate your nervous system. Aim for five breaks a day of two to three minutes to just sit quietly and have a cup of tea or maybe a walk around the block. Somatic breaks (moving or bringing your attention to the body) can be instantly soothing and dial down stress. Try lying on the floor for a few minutes, or wave your hands and legs like seaweed, or count your breaths or stroke the palms of your hands.

Mind your transitions

Transition to home-time from work, or from home to going out in the evening, can be stressful as we are gearing down or up, and whenever we are doing that we go through a temporary dysregulation. Many of us drink to navigate the discomfort of transitions. Give yourself time to settle in the situation and know that the discomfort is temporary.

A sweet bedtime routine

Start to wind down early. After dinner, take a walk or wind down with a TV programme, have a bath with essential oils, make your bedroom a sanctuary, go to bed by 10pm, stay off tech after 8pm and follow the same pattern each night. Explore supplements such as magnesium and passionflower. Self-massage and a weighted blanket may help.

Sleep quality over quantity

Some people instantly see an improvement in their sleep when they stop drinking. However, if you used alcohol to self-medicate for insomnia, it may take time for your sleep to settle. Remember that even if you're sleeping less, you will be having better quality sleep, which is more restorative than passing out and waking up at 3am with a headache and the sweats. If sleep continues to be problematic for you, do get support from your healthcare provider as good sleep is a life source and essential for our wellbeing.

Neurotransmitter hack – serotonin – the mood stabilizer

To counteract the feelings that can come with being tired, feeling low and perhaps depressed this season we are focusing on boosting serotonin, the key hormone that stabilizes our mood, feelings of wellbeing and happiness. It also helps us with our sleeping, eating and digestion. Unlike dopamine, the rewarder, which gives us a hit when we get something we want, serotonin is all about stability and feelings of general wellbeing. Here are some natural ways to boost your serotonin levels:

Brain food

- Dark chocolate
- Avocados
- Cheese, cottage cheese
- Chicken, turkey, salmon
- Eggs
- Granola
- Game/duck
- Yoghurt
- Nuts
- Brown rice

Body food

- Running, biking, walking, swimming
- Chanting
- Meditation

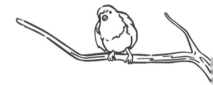

Soul food

- Watching feel good films or box sets with characters we know and love
- Reaching out to people we trust either in real life or in our sober/supportive communities
- Giving a compliment
- Acts of kindness
- Sending yourself flowers
- Self-compassion practice
- Positive affirmations
- Taking a bath

FOR YOUR *Journal*

How does my sleep impact my triggers to drink?

How can I ensure I have a good evening routine?

What does that look like for me?

What do I need to do to help myself sleep well?

What am I going to add in to boost myself when tired and feeling low?

Because I was sober, this week I . . .

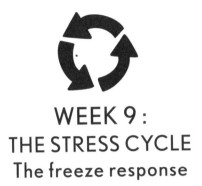

WEEK 9 :
THE STRESS CYCLE
The freeze response

*'Music brings a warm glow to my vision, thawing mind
and muscle from their endless wintering.'*
HARUKI MURAKAMI

The 'freeze' element of the autonomic nervous system's fight/flight/freeze/fawn response
is the ultimate shutdown response that kicks in when an animal feels under inescapable,
imminent threat. This can be seen in the wild when, for example, a gazelle is attacked by
lions and seemingly there is no way out. The animal will go into total shutdown to lessen the
pain of the attack, and play dead in the hope that they will trick the predator and conserve
all the energy they can in order to, if they can get a chance, flee.

In this freeze state, your blood pressure and heart rate drop and blood literally drains into
the core to preserve basic vital functions. This is a deeply intelligent and healthy response
to life-threatening traumatic events and can also happen to humans in the face of shock
or trauma.

However, what was once appropriately adaptive, such as dissociating from an event vastly
beyond your capacity to handle, can become frustratingly maladaptive in later life. If we are
unable to discharge the stress, we become stuck and dysregulated. If we get stuck and have
stored-up survival stress, we are not able to respond appropriately to our environment in the
here and now. There is a fear that if we 'thaw' we will not be safe, so we are literally stuck in
the wrong gear.

According to trauma specialists, there is also a state called 'functional freeze', which means that we are not immobilized in bed or fainting regularly but we live with a quality or sense of being shut down and disconnected. We may experience the freeze response as physical stiffness or heaviness of limbs, decreased heart rate, restricted breathing or holding of the breath, feeling stiff in a certain part of the body and feeling cold or numb.

The freeze response can have a lasting impact on our life – we can zone out, become fearful of trying new things and be indecisive; we might experience a lack of trust and find it difficult to be intimate or form healthy attachments. We have talked before about how alcohol is often used to cope with dysregulation and stress. Dr Gabor Maté, bestselling author and a world-leading clinician in addiction and trauma, believes that all addictions stem from being stuck in one or more of the trauma responses and the dysregulation that brings.

WAYS TO SUPPORT A FREEZE RESPONSE

Here are some self-supporting ways to manage and move out of a freeze response:

1. Grounding, centering and orienting

If you find yourself in the freeze response (or the other stress responses of fight/flight/fawn for that matter), the way back to yourself is to follow these three steps: first, ground yourself by feeling your feet on the ground; then centre yourself by placing your hand on your heart and bringing yourself back in your body, reminding yourself that you are safe, you are loved and you are present; and, finally, orient yourself by noticing where you are right now.

2. Self-soothe with temperature

With the freeze response, our parasympathetic system counterbalances the physical effects of the stress hormones flooding our body by triggering a state of 'freezing' – our heart rate and breathing slows down and we may find that we hold our breath or tense up. You can notice these signs in your body and then literally make sure you warm up to get the blood flowing, with jumpers or sitting by the fire, wearing a big hoody with the hood up, and/or putting on a hat and gloves. Be gentle with yourself: this WILL pass. Wrap yourself in a blanket and treat yourself how you would a frightened child, talk softly to yourself, watch comforting TV, drink tea. Let a loved one know how you are feeling and get some support on board.

3. Shake it out

According to Dr Stephen Porges, expert in polyvagal theory, shaking after a traumatic event to discharge the energy is a healthy response. It is believed that animals in the wild do not experience PTSD because of this ability to shake. So, if you feel yourself in a traumatic state wanting to shake, allow it – it's normal. If you feel you're carrying unprocessed stress from previous situations and are in a safe, appropriate space, allowing your limbs to shake – for example, shaking it out while you dance – can help restore regulation.

FOR YOUR *journal*

Have I ever found myself in the freeze or functional freeze state?

What helps to move me from inaction to action?

What is the best way I can find to ground myself in the present moment?

What is the one thing I can do to look after myself right now?

Who can I reach out to?

Because I was sober, this week I . . .

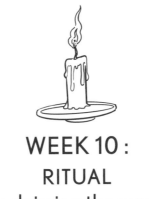

WEEK 10 :
RITUAL
Reclaiming the magic

'And above all, watch with glittering eyes the whole world around you because the greatest secrets are always hidden in the most unlikely places. Those who don't believe in magic will never find it.'
ROALD DAHL

We have touched on the ideas of awe and wonder in springtime, but there is something about magic which feels darker, more mysterious, playful and possibly a bit naughty. With awe and wonder we are blown away by something greater, its beauty and its power – such as the endless rolling in of the waves or the way the birds know how it's time to head south for winter. Magic, on the other hand, conjures up the idea of spells, incantations, tricks and supernatural forces. It makes us clap our hands and wonder if we might get caught.

Magic and the supernatural are sometimes referred to as the things we know that cannot yet be explained by science. We are told there is light and dark magic, although Wiccans believe all magic is grey as we can never completely control the outcome. With magic, we draw on legends and fairy tales. It is the way in which we interact with awe and wonder and use it creatively and intentionally to manifest some change. It's an invocation for some of the power to channel through us in some way. It's inviting the mysteries of life to work, and an attempt to affect how form plays with the unseen. It's a direction of our will in creative and personal ways, an expression of who we are through our own rituals and our own beliefs.

It's a well-known joke in the sober community that at some point, usually in the second year, we go a bit woo. Perhaps you would like to explore the tarot or find you are drawn to reiki and crystals, take up yoga or suddenly fancy a gong bath. We spend such a lot of our time trying to be cool, grown-up and fitting in when we drink, so reclaiming the magic can be about being curious, playful and experimenting again. Ruby Warrington,author of *Spiritual Girl, Material World* and *Sober Curious* believes that being sober and present allows us to have a high vibe and experience life on a deeper and more connected, mystical level.

Spirituality, the supernatural, mystical practices and magic can provide comfort from carrying life's suffering on our shoulders. We fight to protect those we love from pain, and we learn to quieten our yearnings to explore and daydream and create and connect with ourselves and our experience of life in a deeper way. Many people within the sober community connect with some sort of spiritual or magical practice because it helps them to feel less alone. Be it your higher power, god/goddess, the divine feminine or the Universe, sometimes it helps to feel that there is something greater than us out there and ancient wisdoms can provide another layer of meaning in the modern rat-race.

We see magic as accepting all that we are, embracing our 'shadow' (the parts of ourselves that we may not like) and re-friending the whole of ourselves, not being afraid to play and explore, and tapping into our personal power. Magic can be a delicious rediscovery of our own unique experience of the world. Author and artist Dani DiPirro (@positivelypresent) writes about magic in her book *Grow Through It*, describing it as 'the true essence of who you were before the world told you who you "should" be – the parts of yourself that fill you with such wonder that you feel you could spend ages exploring them.' We LOVE that!

How do you embrace your own light and dark magic, your power and your individuality? When we remove a substance that is holding us back, numbing us and dulling our unique brilliance, we stop wasting our own magic. So, embrace your fabulous alcohol-free self, queen, and rock your magic.

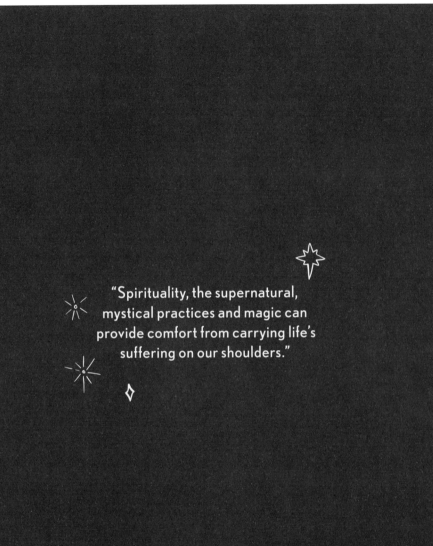

"Spirituality, the supernatural,
mystical practices and magic can
provide comfort from carrying life's
suffering on our shoulders."

FOR YOUR *journal*

Did I believe in magic as a child?

What does magic mean to me?

What are my favourite fairy tales?

How have I reclaimed my magic by fighting for a cause I believe in?

How do I go against the grain?

If I were to cast a spell, what would it be for?

Because I was sober, this week I . . .

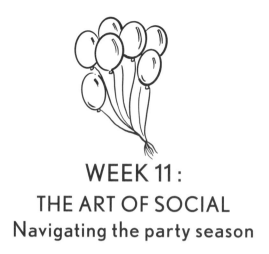

WEEK 11 :
THE ART OF SOCIAL
Navigating the party season

'The world says fit in; the universe says stand out.'
MATSHONA DHLIWAYO

Winter is often a super social season – this may go against our natural rhythms but it has become important in connecting with others and as a way of cheering the spirits in colder months. Earlier in the book we looked at other areas of socializing – our micro-connections, our summer burnout, and JOMO. In winter, we are focusing on going out-out, because Sober Cinderella can go to the ball if she wants to.

Reclaiming this fairy story as a sober metaphor is going to help us get our sparkle and glam on, and having sobriety as your fairy goddess mother means you will never turn into the drunken pumpkin at midnight or any other time. To boss your ball sober you must follow these pieces of advice from your sober fairy goddess mother:

You can go to the ball but be back by midnight (or 10pm if you have had enough)

Most of us neglect that we have a social window of tolerance and use alcohol to push on through longer than we actually want to be somewhere. We shy away from social events because they seem overwhelming or we get triggered to drink, but maybe the clock has chimed and you're still partying after all the fairy godmother's magic has disappeared. What is your social window? Make a plan not to stay one minute over it. Have your carriage waiting and drive it yourself!

A great outfit will do wonders for your confidence

You're sober honey, you deserve it! When we're going sober and social, we like to go all out: nails done, new outfit, hair looking fly, perfume smelling sexy. All these added fantabulous treats afforded by all the money you have saved on booze – yes, queen! Think Diana Ross meets RuPaul – and then some. It's your time to shine, not to shy away. Be proud!

Be prepared – not so much a scout but a badass sober goddess

There is huge power in planning and playing the evening forward right until you leave. What will you wear? Who will you talk to? What will you drink? What will you be proud of? What time will you leave? How will you feel when you wake up in the morning having bossed it? #spoiler – a massive Cheshire cat smile and sense of achievement.
Did you know that if we walk through the steps in our mind, our minds don't entirely differentiate between the thought process and actually having done it, so our brains take this as evidence!

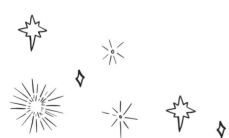

Dance with decorum

Someone once said to us on a sober forum: you can go to the party, you don't have to BE the party. A lot of our socializing was either controlling our drinking (being on edge, not having fun and obsessing over when it would be acceptable for us to have our next drink) or being other people's entertainment – the one who can 'put it back', 'crazy party girl', 'up for it', 'such a laugh when she's p***ed'. In the moment, this made us feel like we had worth – people wanted us around, they thought we were good craic. But where were they at 4am when we woke up with dread? Where were they in the morning when we were being sick? What did they say when we said we were thinking of having a break? Why were we outsourcing our self-esteem to be a performing animal for someone else's laughs, when internally we were suffering? There is ENORMOUS self-affirmation and pride in going to a party and not doing anything that embarrasses you. Of having a sense of feeling like a ballet dancer, straight back, head held high. You have emerged now as a beautiful swan – and watch out fickle friends because this girl can bite.

Keep your special people around you

Our Cinders had her little mice friends with her. You, in turn, can have your sober community with you. Maybe you wear a bracelet that reminds you of milestones. We often say to each other, 'I will have you in my pocket' – as we know that if it all gets too much we can escape to the loo and log on to a sober group and reach out. It's a pretty amazing thing to know that 24/7 somewhere around the world someone will pick that message up and say, 'I got you, what do you need?'

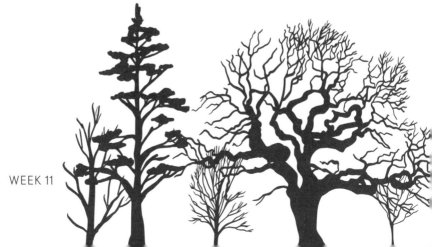

FOR YOUR *journal*

What social events would I like to go to?

What social events can I cancel?

What would be the ideal party for me?

What's my social window?
What would make me feel like a sparkly princess?
(This can be tatts and piercings and all black btw –
sparkle doesn't have to be pink.)

Who makes me feel totally at ease when I am with them?

Who are people who are only fun-time friends?
Is it time to let them go?
Because I was sober, this week I . . .

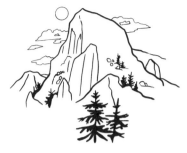

WEEK 12 :
THE SCHOOL OF LIFE
Our future self or meeting the sage

'This life is mine alone. So I have stopped asking people for directions to places they've never been.'
SOCRATES

One of the many gifts of sobriety is a renewed sense of hope and having a future to look forward to, and no matter how old you are you can always benefit from a bit of sage advice from someone even older and wiser! There is a wonderful technique that has long been a favourite of coaches to access some of your inherent wisdom and perspective – the future self-visualization.

Meet your future self (we like to call her your inner sage)

You'll need to put aside 15 minutes with no distractions and have a notebook and pen at the ready, allow your imagination to roam, and be curious as to what comes up when you wander in the playground of the mind.

Step 1. Sit comfortably. Focus on your breathing. Relax and let yourself sink into your chair.

Step 2. Imagine yourself leaving your body, flying up and floating above yourself. Observe yourself and the room you're in as it is in your life today.

Step 3. Fly out of an open window, up into the sky, higher and higher and then imagine you see a beam of sunshine. Drift along this beam, with its warmth surrounding you, forward 20 years to visit the dwelling place of your future wise self, your inner sage.

Step 4. Observe where she lives. Is it town or country? What country?

Step 5. Go to the door and knock. She answers. What does she look like, what is she wearing, how do you feel seeing her?

Step 6. What is her home like? What colours has she decorated with? Is it modern? Is it traditional?

Step 7. Your inner sage offers you something to eat and a drink. What is it? Where do you sit? Does she have any animals?

Step 8. You have a conversation with her. What advice does she give you? What does she want you to remember? To focus on? Ask her: what do I need to get from where I am to where you are? Ask her anything you would like to know.

Step 9. When it is time to leave, she gives you a gift; she doesn't explain it and asks you to open it when you're back in your current life. You thank her and fly back up into the sky. Then follow the warm soft sunbeam back down into your current life.

Step 10. Bring your focus back to your breathing. Take a moment to wriggle your fingers and toes, give yourself a hug, pat at your arms and notice where you are to orient yourself. Take a moment and then open your journal when you are ready to make some notes about your conversation with your inner sage.

As you go about your daily life and make decisions, if you're feeling stressed or worried about anything, chat to your inner sage, give her a name, ask her for advice. 'What would my wisest self do right now?' is a powerful question that helps us to pause and get in alignment with what we want rather than just reacting to life's events without thinking.

You may like to read what you have written out loud and record it on your phone to play it back. You could even have someone else read it to you. You can also visit our website at lovesober.com for a free audio file to talk you through this visualization.

When you need to bring yourself back to your true north and realign with your sober values, check in with your inner sage. What does she do with her free time? How does she talk, how does she handle difficult situations, how does she care for herself? What are her great loves?

My sage self lives in a fabulous beach house on her own on the Pacific Coast somewhere. She is a bit like Meryl Streep in *Mamma Mia*. Whenever I call on her, I feel more balanced and get a sense of perspective, which calms feelings of panic or worry for me. She basically tells me to chill and that whatever I am het up about doesn't actually matter in the long run, which is super helpful when you are a professional catastrophist like me. KATE

It brings enormous comfort to be able to check in with my wise sage future self. When I met her, I knew she didn't want to be a drunk grandma being put to bed by her kids with her grandkids watching; she wanted to be inspirational, steady, available and doing things like trekking in mountains and paddleboarding with rad self-affirming tattoos. MANDY

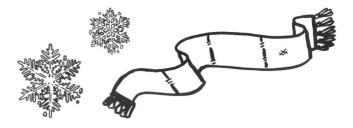

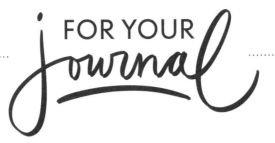

FOR YOUR Journal

What did she tell me?
What did I learn from meeting her?
What were her answers to my questions?
How did I feel when I met her?

What are my priorities now?
Close my eyes again and imagine opening the present she gave me.
What is it?

What is the significance of this gift?
How can it guide me?
Because I was sober, this week I . . .

WEEK 13 :
TOOLS FOR GREATER REFLECTION
Journaling

*'There is no greater agony than bearing
an untold story inside you.'*
MAYA ANGELOU

Journaling is a brilliant reflective practice which helps increase self-awareness and emotional intelligence. By checking in regularly with ourselves we can process blocked emotions and check progress toward our goals.

Moon journaling – using the new moon to set intentions and the full moon as a time to reflect – allows more time between entries and can provide an overarching sense of transition and progress by using a monthly rhythm. Try to get outside and look at the moon and, when you do this, notice as much as you can – the full low Harvest Moons, the icy winter moons, how the clouds move across the moon and maybe spot a moon rainbow.

The moon is also seen as the female energy counterpart to the sun's male fiery energy, linked with dreams and intuition, and so is a natural guide in cultivating a mindful, cyclical practice.

Full moons throughout the year

Each month's full moon has an evocative name, many first coined by indigenous North Americans many years ago. In the Southern Hemisphere, the names are simply switched to allow for the opposite seasons, so January's Wolf Moon is seen in July.

January: Wolf Moon	July: Buck Moon
February: Snow Moon	August: Sturgeon Moon
March: Worm Moon	September: Harvest Moon
April: Pink Moon	October: Hunter's Moon
May: Flower Moon	November: Beaver Moon
June: Strawberry Moon	December: Cold Moon

The Three Parts of the Moon Cycle – creating a journal practice

First, get organized by using a dated diary, bullet journal or perennial calendar. Mark out the moon cycles, full moon and new moons for the year. You might like to mark the names of the moons above and explore these for greater reflection and creativity when journaling.

New Moon intentions

Ask yourself: What do I want to focus on this cycle? What new ideas are forming? What needs care and attention? What does my heart desire? What will I cultivate? What is my secret wish? Note your new moon mood, energy levels and sleep rhythm.

Full Moon reflections

Ask yourself: Where am I now in terms of the intentions I set? Has anything shifted or improved? What can I let go of? If you love to work creatively, ask the moon for an unexpected gift. Note your full moon mood, energy levels and sleep patterns.

The Dark Moon

This is the end of the previous moon cycle. It is the moment in time where we are absorbing everything that we learned in the previous moon cycle and is an opportunity to do a final audit before we begin the new cycle. It's time to rest, pause and integrate before we set new moon intentions.

Ask yourself: What memories did I make in this closing moon cycle? What challenges did I face? How can I grow from them? What goals can I reboot and how can I move a step closer to these goals?

The dark moon is also a powerful time to connect with your Shadow – the parts of yourself you don't like very much or your uncomfortable emotions. It's an opportunity to give compassion to those hurt parts of yourself.

Ask yourself: What came up for me this month, what did I struggle with? What frustrations and irritations were noteworthy? What lessons did I learn? What wisdom am I taking forward into the next moon cycle?

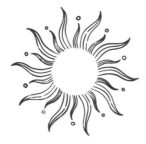

WINTER SOLSTICE
Ritual and reflection

'The darkest hour comes before the dawn.'
PROVERB

The winter solstice is the day when the hours of daylight are at their shortest. This has been marked throughout history and is still celebrated worldwide as the moment when the days start lengthening. In the UK, at Stonehenge the druids still gather, while in Brighton there is the festival of Burning of the Clocks. In Iran, the winter solstice is celebrated as Shab-e Yalda, while in China it is the festival of Dongzhi; there is Inti Raymi in Peru, and the festival of Soyal celebrated by the Hopi people of Arizona.

This idea of the darkest hour or day has a special resonance for sober people. We can liken it to the 'rock bottom' if we have had one, or that moment when we said, 'enough is enough.' It is in that moment of surrender to what is, when new possibility is born. This is the winter solstice moment. Our lowest points are like inner winter solstices, which are often our biggest life lessons and the welcome mat to healing.

When we are in them, we feel like there is no light and wonder how we will cope. We wonder how we are ever going to climb out of the pit, but midwinter reminds us that the darkest hour comes before the dawn, and sobriety reminds us that all things shall pass. So we can seek comfort in knowing that we are in the family of things – we are one with nature, not separate from it, and part of those greater cycles, and we know that lighter days are coming. We light fires, connect with others and celebrate what has been and what is to come to keep us cheerful and keep our spirits up.

The message of the solstice is: tomorrow is lighter, and the next day even lighter! Other days may be dark, but they are not as dark as the darkest. Autumn was rewriting our story by releasing things that were holding us back. Now we rest, before asking, 'What are the things we want to reorganize and restore?' before the wheel turns once more and we prepare, thankfully, for another journey around the sun.

After the rest and the dark, we turn toward the light of the dawn of a new spring and a new cycle begins . . .

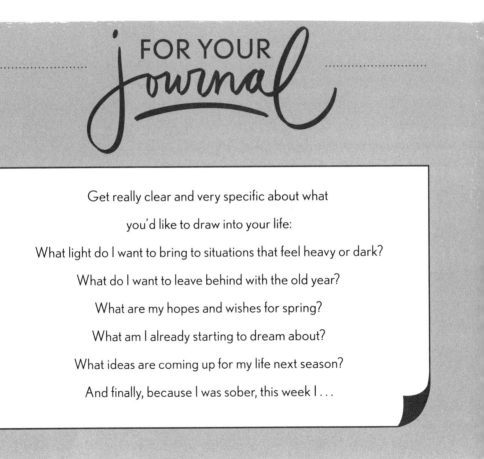

FOR YOUR *Journal*

Get really clear and very specific about what

you'd like to draw into your life:

What light do I want to bring to situations that feel heavy or dark?

What do I want to leave behind with the old year?

What are my hopes and wishes for spring?

What am I already starting to dream about?

What ideas are coming up for my life next season?

And finally, because I was sober, this week I . . .

FINAL THOUGHTS

We wrote this book with the backdrop of one of the most incredibly stressful years for us both personally, and the irony is not lost on us. For much of this year, we sat on either side of the English Channel on Zoom, due to a fractured, Brexited Europe and being in the midst of a global pandemic, going 'WTF?'. We cycled through periods of burnout, perimenopause, illness, family crises and ALL.THE.THINGS. We have had to practise the tools in this book as we asked for help, told the truth to ourselves and others, learned to say 'No' and forced ourselves to rest. The one constant was that neither of us drank, as one thing we both knew deep in our souls is that if we had it would have been catastrophic. Such is the power of the sober toolkit. The message for us is that whatever happens, it's always better to be sober and we are forever grateful for the choice we made to choose ourselves over alcohol.

It was our intention in writing *Love Your Sober Year* to work with the seasons, with stories and with science as a framework to heal body, mind and soul. If we understand brain science, habits and our nervous systems we can be equipped enough to be intentional, manage triggers and change our behaviour. We needed the calming elements of nature to give us perspective, the creativity and fun we find in exploring in stories and metaphors to excite us, and a hefty dose of science and psychology to satisfy our inquisitive minds.

At Love Sober, we coach women individually and in our group programmes. Using the universal framework of the Panarchic theory, the seasons of our world and our lives, we honed our holistic R4 Balance Method to create the perpetual cycle of Restore, Reignite, Rewrite and Rest. We have illustrated in this book that as we cycle through the seasons as the Earth turns and we face our lives' transitions, we must return to these wisdoms over and over, as is the cyclical journey as women in sobriety.

We return to REST in our lives to gain clarity, RESTORE to heal and learn, REIGNITE for our passion for living and REWRITE to reframe our story.

Although it was our intention to write an engaging and inspiring guide to seasonal sober living and journaling, and to be a comforting and uplifting companion, *Love Your Sober Year* has a serious side to it. On a personal note, the reason we drank has its roots in our individual experiences of trauma over the years combined with the potent addictive nature of alcohol. Even if you have not experienced a shocking traumatic event or had childhood trauma, the dysregulation from chronically busy lives and from being women in a patriarchal society is inherently traumatic because of its inequalities. We would like to also acknowledge the trauma of othering that happens daily for the LGBTQ+ community, people of colour, those living with disabilities and the neurodiverse, too. The systemic rejection of the feminine nature which is innate in all of us regardless of any assigned gender has also led to toxic masculinity, underfunded services for women's health and a society that is so stuck 'doing' all the time, we have forgotten how to 'be'.

The Dalai Lama is quoted as saying 'Western women will save the world,' and although it seems like a stretch (sweating head emoji), the ability to be heard and connect with each other via tech has never been greater, and watching young women like Greta Thunburg, Emma Watson and Amanda Gorman shining their lights and effecting change in the world certainly gives us hope. Interestingly, science is coming full circle and the labs of Berkeley and Harvard are backing up the old wisdoms of meditation and the benefits to mind, body and soul of 'feminine' qualities such as kindness, compassion with metadata and PET scans. The science of the autonomic nervous system and polyvagal theory confirms the importance of nurture and connection with other humans in terms of health and longevity, and the fact we survive together not apart.

Against the backdrop of climate change and the planet's depleting resources, there has never been a better time to slow down, take stock and really embrace the principles of sustainable living to heal the planet and ourselves – and if we start in ways that we can change and control, we can have hope.

We wish for you the joy of a grounded, healthy and sustainable life, no longer hampered by the damaging effects of alcohol. We wish for you a toolkit so full you can always call on yourself, and joyful connections to know you can call on others to help. We wish you clarity to know that booze is a liar and a thief of joy and we wish you your own unique, full experience, as Mary Oliver would say, of your 'one wild and precious life'.

As you move forward, check back in with these seasons when you need inspiration. Use the journal questions for self-reflection, time and again – they are evergreen. Come and say hi to us at Love Sober. Stay mindful, stay connected and always remember to look up at the moon and the stars, at the beauty of architecture, at the trees and at blue sky, and own your place in the 'family of things'.

With love, Kate and Mandy xxxx

RESOURCES

Join us at Love Sober www.lovesober.com. Reach out for further support at
She Recovers® – www.sherecovers.org

Recommended reading

Brach, T (2020). *Radical Compassion*. Rider Publishing.

Brewer, J (2018). *The Craving Mind*. Yale University Press.

Brown, B (2017). *Braving the Wilderness & The Gifts of Imperfections*. Vermillion Publishing.

Chapple, S (2019). *The Sober Survival Guide*. Elevator Digital Ltd.

Chapple, S (2021). *How to Heal Your Inner Child*. Sheldon Press.

Clear, J (2018). *Atomic Habits*. Random House Business.

Cyrulnik, B (2009). *Resilience*. Penguin.

Dana, D (2020). *Polyvagal Exercises for Safety & Connection*. WW Norton & Company.

Dipirro, D (2020). *Grow Through It*. LOM ART.

Duhigg, C (2013). *The Power of Habit*. Random House Books.

Gooch, M (2021). *The Sober Girl Society*. Bantam Press.

Haidt, J (2021). *The Happiness Hypothesis*. Random House Business.

Hardy, J (2017). *The Self-Care Project*. Orion Spring.

Hardy, J (2021). *Making Space*. Experiment.

Hepola, S (2016). *Blackout*. Two Roads.

Johnston, A (2015). *Drink*. Fourth Estate Ltd.

Le'Nise (2022). *You Can Have a Better Period*. Watkins Publishing.

Manners, M & Baily, K (2020). *Love Yourself Sober*. Trigger Publishing.

Maté, G (2018). *In the Real of Hungry Ghosts*. Vermillion.

Mohr, T (2015). *Playing Big*. Arrow Publishing.

May, K (2020). *Wintering*. Rider.

Nagoski, E & A (2019). *Burnout*. Vermillion Publishing.

Pooley, C (2018). *The Sober Diaries*. Coronet.

Pope, A & Wurlitzer, S (2017). *Wild Power*. Hay House UK.

Porter, W (2015). *Alcohol Explained*. CreateSpace.

Rocca, L (2013). *The Sober Revolution*. Headline Accent.

Rubin, G (2018). *The Four Tendencies*. Two Roads Publishing.

Russel, B (2020). *How to Be Hopeful*. Elliot & Thompson Ltd.

Seligman, M (2011). *Flourish*. Nicholas Brealey Publishing.

Sommerville, A (2021). *How to be a boss at Ageing*. Thread.

Trimpey, J (1996). *Rational Recovery*. Gallery Books.

Van de Kolk, B (2015). *The Body Keeps the Score*. Penguin.

Walker, P (2013). *Complex PTSD From Surviving to Thriving*. CreateSpace.

Walker, R (2016). *A Happier Hour*. Mod by Dom.

Winfrey, O & Perry, B (2021). *What Happened to You?* Bluebird.

ACKNOWLEDGEMENTS

WITH THANKS TO:

Our wonderful families – our husbands Dave & Paul and our kids William & Ella and Matilda & Albert.

The brilliant team at Welbeck Publishing – our publisher Jo Lal, our awesome editor Becky Miles and our agent Jane Graham-Maw at Graham Maw Christie Agency.

The sober movement on Instagram and the Love Sober Community.

Le'nise Brothers, Alexandra Pope and Sjanie Hugo Wurlitzer at Red School (www.redschool.net) for their insight and activism around menstrual health.

Lou Lebenz & Mel Curtis of Trauma Thrivers and Irene Lyon for their expertise and knowledge of trauma and the biology of stress.

The brilliant supportive team at the Coaching Academy.

If you are interested in becoming a coach and would like to train with us, please get in touch:

www.the-coaching-academy.com/coaching/addictive-behaviours-coaching

ABOUT US

Welbeck Balance publishes books dedicated to changing lives. Our mission is to deliver life-enhancing books to help improve your wellbeing so that you can live your life with greater clarity and meaning, wherever you are on life's journey. Our Trigger books are specifically devoted to opening up conversations about mental health and wellbeing.

Welbeck Balance and Trigger are part of the Welbeck Publishing Group – a globally recognized independent publisher. Welbeck are renowned for our innovative ideas, production values and developing long-lasting content. Our books have been translated into over 30 languages in more than 60 countries around the world.

If you love books, then join the club and sign up to our newsletter for exclusive offers, extracts, author interviews and more information.

www.welbeckpublishing.com   www.triggerhub.org

 welbeckpublish   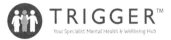 Triggercalm
welbeckpublish   Triggercalm
welbeckuk   Triggercalm

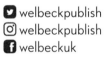

WELBECK
BALANCE

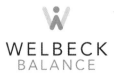 TRIGGER™
Your Specialist Mental Health & Wellbeing Hub